Activities with Developmentally Disabled Elderly and Older Adults

M. Jean Keller
Editor

The Haworth Press
New York • London

Activities with Developmentally Disabled Elderly and Older Adults has also been published as *Activities, Adaptation & Aging,* Volume 15, Numbers 1/2 1990.

The Haworth Press, Inc., 10 Alice Street, Binghamton, NY 13904-1580
EUROSPAN/Haworth, 3 Henrietta Street, London WC2E 8LU England

Library of Congress Cataloging-in-Publication Data

Activities with developmentally disabled elderly and older adults / M. Jean Keller, editor.
    p. cm.
    "Has also been published as Activities, adaptation & aging, volume 15, numbers 1/2, 1990" – T.p. verso.
    Includes bibliographical references.
    ISBN 1-56024-092-X (alk. paper)
    1. Developmentally disabled aged – Rehabilitation. 2. Art therapy for the aged. 3. Recreational therapy for the aged. I. Keller, M. Jean.
    [DNLM: 1. Mental Retardation – in old age. 2. Mental Retardation – rehabilitation. 3. Recreation. W1 AC9802 v. 15 no. 1/2 / WM 308 A188]
RC953.8.A75A27 1990
618.97′6858803 – dc20
DNLM/DLC
for Library of Congress

                        168149   90-5310
                                               CIP

Also published as ISBN: 1-56024-174-8 (pbk.)

Activities
with Developmentally
Disabled Elderly
and Older Adults

CONTENTS

ABOUT THE EDITOR

M. Jean Keller, EdD, CTRS, is Associate Professor in the Recreation and Leisure Studies Program at the University of North Texas. Dr. Keller has extensive experience, both academic and professional, in therapeutic recreation, developmental disabilities, and gerontology.

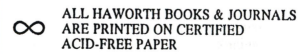

Introduction

M. Jean Keller

The older adult population with developmental disabilities (DD) continues to grow rapidly; yet, little is known about their needs and interests. As the literature and research was reviewed related to elderly persons with DD and recreation activities, there was also a noticeable void. As such, it is especially pleasing that this text, *Activities with Developmentally Disabled Elderly and Older Adults*, has been developed for publication to address this needed topic. The purpose of this text is to focus on the growing number of older people with developmental disabilities and how to effectively plan and deliver activities with them.

It was satisfying and rewarding to receive manuscripts concerning diverse issues, services, and programs from researchers, educators, and practitioners representing varied disciplines. Clearly no one activity or service delivery strategy is right for all older persons with developmental disabilities in different settings. The chapters presented in this text demonstrate the diversity which makes serving a growing number of older individuals with DD both challenging and rewarding.

The lead chapter, "Activities and Adaptation: A Call for Innovations to Serve Aging Adults with Developmental Disabilities," highlights the characteristics of this population and challenges activity professionals to seek innovative program strategies to appropriately serve individuals with DD. Hawkins and Kultgen discuss companionship/friendship, physical functioning, and retirement adjustment as three major quality of life themes that confront older adults who have lived with lifelong disabling conditions. Riddick and Keller explain how a continuum of recreational activities is needed to provide meaningful experiences to elders with developmental disabilities. Recreation professionals are invited and encouraged to assist older adults with DD acquire the knowledge and skills necessary to pursue recreational activities that are appropriate to their abilities, interests, and age level and which will foster their physical, social, mental, and/or emotional well-being. "Therapeutic Recreation Programming for Older Adults with Developmental Disabilities" presents an approach to designing therapeutic recreation programs. Carter and Foret share a training model to facilitate coordination among caregivers and professionals as activity plans are developed for aging adults with DD. In order to provide meaningful activities with older people who are developmentally disabled, appropriate needs assessment instruments are required. See, Ellis, Spellman, and Cress describe a survey instrument used to gain information about the needs of elderly persons with DD living in rural areas and how the survey results were used in program planning both for the agency and individuals.

Specific programs and services that are age appropriate and foster creative expression and positive self-esteem for elders with DD are often unavailable. The next three chapters focus on programming with older adults with developmental disabilities. Harlan offers a model program based on the concept of art as therapy. Edelson likewise promotes the value of art and craft activities as meaningful avocational experiences. Both Harlan and Edelson address issues of program design, implementation, and evaluation related to the use of art with elderly persons who are developmentally disabled. Developing positive social and communication skills may present great challenges for persons who are aged and developmentally disabled. Yet, as Segal describes these skills are essential to life functioning and proposes the use of expressive arts (music, art and movement) within group settings to develop and enhance communication and socialization skills.

An increasing number of older adults with DD are living in community settings and in need of community recreation services. A rationale for development of integrated recreation programs is discussed by Wilhite, Keller, and Nicholson. An interdisciplinary model of recreation integration is highlighted and illustrated through a case study of an older individual with DD. "Sharing Activities — The Oneida County A.R.C. Cornhill Senior Center Integration Project," by Zimpel describes an integration process of older persons with DD with their nondisabled peers. The dynamics of how and why integration of older persons with and without disabilities can be accomplished are highlighted.

The concluding chapter, "Aging, Developmental Disabilities and Leisure: Policy and Service Delivery Issues," takes us back to the beginning of this special text. Tedrick deducts that presently there are more questions than answers surrounding cooperative initiatives involving DD systems and aging service networks. While we have only begun to scratch the surface, we have begun to address issues of activities and adaptations needed to better serve older adults with developmental disabilities. Practitioners, educators, researchers, policy makers, and each of us are challenged to begin to seek answers and solutions to questions and issues related to providing meaningful activities with a growing population with unique needs and interests.

For this special text every effort was made to attract a wide variety of authors, share innovative and creative strategies for programming activities with older adults with DD, and stimulate interest and continued support for recreation program development and implementation among developmental disability and aging service systems. My sincere thanks are extended to all who submitted manuscripts for consideration; this text would have been impossible without your contributions. The manuscript reviewers, Paul D. Cotten, George A. Foelker, Jr., John W. Gibson, Barbara Hawkins, John Keiter, Phyllis Kultgen, Susan Lynch, Ann M. Rancourt, Jenny C. Overeynder, Esther Lee Pederson, and Ruth Roberts were a delight to work with and their dedication and competent work was respected and appreciated. Dr. Barbara A. Hawkins, Assistant Professor of Recreation at Indiana University, and Director of the Program on Aging and Developmental Disabilities, I. U. Institute for the Study of Developmental Disabilities, assisted in the identification of reviewers and authors and offered excellent suggestions and recommendations to the editor. Her interest and support enhanced this special text. Dr. Susan D. Hudson, Professor and Coordinator of Recreation and Leisure Studies, reviewed the final version of this text. Her assistance enriched this work significantly. Ms. Susan E. Lynch, M.S., a doctoral candidate in therapeutic recreation at

Texas Women's University, provided editorial assistance and coordination. Additionally, she prepared book reviews of current texts related to aging adults with DD. Her assistance was sincerely appreciated.

Many thanks to Phyllis M. Foster, ACTIVITIES, ADAPTATION & AGING Editor, Karen Lee, Special Issues Coordinator, and the editorial staff for their support of this endeavor. Appreciation is extended to the University of North Texas Department of Kinesiology, Health Promotion, and Recreation for the support and resources devoted to this effort of the editor. Finally, sincere thanks to you, the reader, who hopefully will find the information shared within this text useful and beneficial to expanding and improving activity services and delivery strategies for older adults with developmental disabilities.

Chapter 1

Activities and Adaptation: A Call for Innovations to Serve Aging Adults with Developmental Disabilities

Barbara A. Hawkins
Phyllis B. Kultgen

SUMMARY. Aging in people with developmental disabilities has emerged as a new area of concern within the past two decades. Little is known, however, about the influence of aging for this population, especially in terms of planning and delivering appropriate activities. This article briefly overviews characteristics of the population. It further describes exemplary program strategies from three areas: companionship, physical activity, and retirement preparation. Challenges to activity professionals are suggested.

INTRODUCTION

During the past two decades, service providers in the developmental disabilities (DD) system have become increasingly aware of the aging phenomenon as it has begun to significantly impact this

---

Barbara A. Hawkins, ReD, is Assistant Professor of Recreation at Indiana University, and Director of the Program on Aging and Developmental Disabilities, I.U. Institute for the Study of Developmental Disabilities. Dr. Hawkins serves as Associate Editor for the AALR/ATR *Annual in Therapeutic Recreation* and the *Therapeutic Recreation Journal*, and is Author/Editor of *Aging and Developmental Disabilities – A Training Inservice Package*. Phyllis B. Kultgen, PhD, is Director of Training for the Program on Aging and Developmental Disabilities at the Institute for the Study of Developmental Disabilities – Indiana University. Dr. Kultgen has authored several training manuals in the area of aging and DD, and is a contributing author to *Aging and Developmental Disabilities – A Training Inservice Package*.

5

population group. At a recent national symposium, Ray (1990) pinpointed this area as one of ten top trends and issues for leisure service providers in the decade to come. The increased attention, within the past few years, by recreation professionals to this group holds promise for the development of needed activity programs that can be adapted for the dual phenomenon of aging and developmental disabilities (Benz, Halpern, & Close, 1986; Boyd & James, 1990; Hawkins, 1987 & 1989a; Rancourt, 1989 & 1990).

Not only is a greying of the population a trend for the larger society but also a new direction for people who have been developmentally challenged throughout their lives. This changing course in demography is particularly poignant in light of the historical context for people who have mental retardation or some other developmental disability. Formerly, for these people, life expectancy was typically short and tenuous. In more recent decades, as treatment models have emphasized habilitation and humane treatment, people with developmental disabilities are surviving into adulthood and many are reaching later maturity. With the emergence of significant numbers of aging and aged adults with developmental disabilities has come the need for new information, collaborative efforts between the aging and DD networks, and trained professionals from both service sectors to deliver appropriate programs.

This chapter provides an overview of the background information on the older DD population. Program strategies that have been developed and are being evaluated will be presented. Research and program innovations that are needed will be suggested with some implications drawn for activity professionals.

POPULATION BACKGROUND

It has been estimated that the size of the older adult population with developmental disabilities for the nation in 1980 was around 200,000 (Janicki, Seltzer, Krauss & Gaetani, 1989). Problems with the estimation of size have been widely discussed in the literature and include the lack of reliable national studies on which to establish age adjusted prevalence rates as a concern (Jacobson, Sutton, & Janicki, 1985; Janicki, Krauss, & Seltzer, 1987; Lubin & Kiely, 1985; Rose & Janicki, 1986). Existing prevalence rates have varied from .34% to 3% (DiGiovanni, 1978; Rose & Janicki, 1986) for the population. Based on the 1980 census, these rates yield a very broad range in potential size from 200,000 to 1.4 million people. An accurate, as opposed to estimated, prevalence rate that is adjusted distinctly for age is needed; particularly, as it will provide a more accurate assessment of the population size.

In spite of the problems associated with determining the actual size of this group, numerous state-level assessment and planning efforts have been made in recent years (Hawkins & Eklund, 1989, 1990). These studies have done much to describe the needs and attributes of the population. They serve as a benchmark in the planning and public policy development process that usually accompanies population groups that have the need for government-sponsored human services. These services include health care, living arrangements, rehabilitative and habilitative care, advocacy and protection, and other support services such as case coordination and transportation.

The identified service areas (Hawkins & Eklund, 1990) that aging and older people with developmental disabilities typically need include those that are listed in Figure 1. These services relate to both the aging process and the presence of developmental disability, and may be exacerbated by these circumstances in combination.

To better understand service needs, it will be helpful to review characteristics of aging and older adults with developmental disabilities. Most of the research on aging processes in people with DD, however, has been done on people who have mental retardation as their primary diagnosis (Janicki, Seltzer, Krauss, & Gaetani, 1989). There remains a dearth of research information about aging processes in persons who have other lifelong disabling conditions such as cerebral palsy, epilepsy, and autism. Thus, it is important to keep in mind that much of what follows pertains to people with mental retardation.

Health, Physical, and Behavioral Characteristics

The research evidence on physical functioning and health status for people with mental retardation who are aging presents a mixed

FIGURE 1. Service Needs of Aging/Aged Adults with DD

Health Care Services: Routine geriatric multidimensional functional assessment; disease prevention/intervention & preventive health care such as screenings and treatment in denture/oral health care, vision and hearing, hypertension, cancer, diabetes, etc; mental health and counseling care.

Residential Services: Planning for and transition to residential environment that supports aging-related change while promoting aging in place.

Day Programming Services: Employment related activities; retirement including pre-retirement preparation, leisure activity development, meaningful community role; redefined day training to focus on habilitative, rehabilitative, and maintenance goals.

Support Services: Service coordination/case management across aging and DD including planning for financial, residential, and guardianship issues in late life; transportation; family support, referral, education, and counseling; self-advocacy preparation.

picture. Some studies suggest little difference between aging people with and without mental retardation on health status (Anderson, Lakin, Bruininks, and Hill, 1987). Krauss and Seltzer (1986) found that older adults had fewer medical problems than younger adults with mental retardation with the exception of sensory impairments. However, Janicki and MacEachron (1984) found that the older adults used medical services more than did younger adults. These conflicting findings may be confounded by the place of residence (institutional, group home, natural family), accessible medical services, geographic location (rural, urban), or selected attributes of the cohort studied.

In spite of conflicting results among both cross sectional and longitudinal studies on functional status, contemporary viewpoints support observable declines in motoric and sensory function apparent in people in their fifties. Other behavioral skills, however, are maintained and may even continue to improve (i.e., daily living skills and intellectual functions) until the seventh decade. The severity of mental retardation or developmental disability, as well as cohort effects (i.e., long periods of institutionalization), may influence the degree of decline and thus, overall life expectancy (Janicki & Jacobson, 1986; Krauss & Seltzer, 1986; Eyman & Widaman, 1987).

While design weaknesses are evident in the current available research (Seltzer, 1985), developmentally challenged people who live into older adulthood do not appear to be drastically different in their physical, health, and behavioral needs from other elderly people. The implication from this finding is that many existing programs and service strategies hold promise for meeting the needs for this population group in terms of daily health, physical, and behavioral functions.

Social Function and Support Characteristics

For the general population of elderly people, social support and social activities revolve around informal caregivers (i.e., family members, neighbors, friends) and the senior services network. For aging and older people with developmental disabilities, this pattern is markedly different.

Most elderly people with developmental disabilities no longer live at home, nor do they have spouses and adult children who can provide social support for them. While Seltzer (1989a, 1989b) and Krauss (1989) have reported preliminary evidence on the differences between the support networks of aging adults with mental retardation compared to the general population, these findings are some of the first to be produced in the research arena.

Little is known about the patterns and changes in sibling involvement over the lifecourse of aging adults with DD. The social relationships that do exist for this population tend to consist of co-residents in congregate residential facilities, friends at work or day activity centers, and paid caregivers (Rinck & Kultgen, 1987). The lack of a stable social support network is one of the most troubling concerns of older adults with DD.

Also, little is known about the retirement and leisure activity involvement of members of this population group. The role of recreational and leisure activities as core components of a habilitation plan, particularly as vocational objectives lessen in prominence, is an area for research. Ascertaining needs, interests and functional skills that promote free time use, as well as maintain other functional and behavioral skills, may well be one of the most critical areas for program development. Some research evidence (Hawkins, 1989) suggests that older adults with mental retardation have a wide range of leisure interests but may be constrained by the lack of friends or equipment needed to pursue those interests. Additional constraints include the lack of instruction in how to perform preferred activities and lack of choice in selecting activities.

Clearly, in terms of social function and activity involvement, the lives of elderly people with DD are not parallel to the general elderly population (Foelker & Luke, 1989). Older adults with DD, however, do experience feelings of grief and adjustment to changes in their own functioning as well as to other losses (i.e., death of friends, family) that are common in later life stages (Menolascino & Potter, 1989). Residential relocation (i.e., transition trauma), removal of work related social networks, the lack of a family support network, and the variable presence of a well developed pattern of leisure activity involvement may heighten awareness of vulnerabilities associated with being developmentally challenged and living a long life.

EXEMPLARY PROGRAM STRATEGIES

Based on known vulnerabilities for people who are old with DD, three broad areas in which exemplary programs have been developed will be discussed. These three areas encompass companionship/friendship, physical functioning, and retirement adjustment. Programming strategies in these three areas are innovative because they address the specific concerns of older adults who have lived with lifelong disabling conditions that have constrained the development of normalized lifestyles and patterns. Thus, innovations in these programs are reflective of important needs for aging adults with DD and represent creative solutions to a changed focus in habilitation planning. Each of these areas are special areas in terms of their contribution to adjustment, overall health, functioning, and quality of life in older adulthood for people who have DD.

Companionship/Friendship

In response to the constricted informal social support networks of older persons with developmental disabilities, a number of demonstration companionship/friendship projects emerged during the decade of the 1980s. The aim of such programs has been to expand opportunities for both community participation and peer companionship. The emergent model projects are considered innovative because of the emphasis given to friendship pairing between an elder from the local community and an older person with a disability.

The Community Access Program, originating in Akron, Ohio under a grant from the Joseph P. Kennedy, Jr. Foundation (Stroud and Sutton, 1988), uses peer companions, either volunteer or employed, to accompany older persons with mental retardation into the community. These "senior friends" introduce people with disabilities to the wide range of leisure and recreational activity options that exist beyond the boundaries of their sheltered residential setting. Community activities in this model may include participation in specifically designated senior activities (i.e., senior centers, golden age clubs, senior exercise) or in community-wide leisure and recreational options.

The Companion Program developed across mid-Missouri through funding from the Administration on Aging (Kultgen, Rinck, Calkins and Intagliata, 1986) uses volunteers from local senior centers to act as companion hosts to mature adults with developmental disabilities. The companion pairs interact during the noon meal at a senior meal-site and during activities such as bingo, dancing, song-fest and so forth. In this program, interaction is limited to the senior site. Both model projects have the short term objective of enlarging the friendship networks of the participants and the long term goal of increasing functional independence.

A number of similar programs, based on the common assumption that affiliation with one's own age group is a developmental tendency among older persons (Havighurst, 1972), have emerged along with the models described above. For example, integration into the normalized setting of a generic senior meal or recreation site is a common endeavor across the country. Some of those efforts avoid identifying the older person with mental retardation as disabled. It is felt that when persons are introduced as clients of the MR/DD system, the "red flag" goes up and the general membership may refuse to accept them. Recognizing the low ratio of staff to participants at typical meal and recreation sites, DD system advocates of the anonymous approach recommend bolstering the senior center staff with the presence of an additional staff person underwritten by the responsible MR/DD agency. This staff person also remains anonymous but is on hand to tend to unanticipated needs that may arise as a result of added numbers of attendants at the site.

In the companion programs described above, very few persons with disabilities are in attendance at any one time. When the anonymous approach is used, the number of persons with special needs may be greater. Although space restrictions preclude descriptions of the great variety of emerging programs aimed at community integration for the purposes of enlarging friendship networks, promoting functional independence, and enhancing quality of life, it is safe to conclude that a trend toward integration programs for older adults with mental retardation has been established.

Physical Fitness/Activity

The concern for health, wellness and physical fitness for all people has steadily grown in recent years. These concerns take on special significance for aging adults with DD for several reasons. Martz (1989) pointed out that adults with DD are "less apt to spontaneously complain or to call attention to abnormal functions" (p. 4). Routine care of feet, dental, skin, vision, and hearing also have been cited as lacking for this population (Buehler, Smith, & Fifield, 1985; Martz, 1989). Physical activity as a key component to the overall promotion of health among the elderly has been recognized as equally important for older adults with DD (Clements, 1989; Engeman & Pederson, 1989; Hawkins, 1989b).

Engeman and Pederson (1989) have implemented a demonstration program at the University Affiliated Cincinnati Center for Developmental Disorders. A supervised physical exercise protocol as recommended by the American College of Sports Medicine and American Heart Association served as the foundation for the program. In addition, a special rowing component that had previously been developed in Cincinnati was used to test the effects of routine physical fitness on a variety of health and behavioral measures. This project also used nutrition education to complete its health/fitness promoting program. This project demonstrated support for previous findings that have shown the benefits of supervised physical activity and fitness programs for adults with DD (Allen, 1980; Schurrer, Brammell, & Weltman, 1985).

As the Public Health Service moves into the next decade with its year 2000 health objectives for the nation, physical fitness for older adults is a targeted area. The same concern for elderly people with DD is appropriate and of heightened significance given the tendency for these people to live sedentary lives with limited leisure skills necessary to promote health and well-being. In concert with the tendency to observe declines in gross motor skills as early as the fifth decade, increased efforts to enhance physical fitness across the life span and into the senior years takes on added importance. Activity programs that offer motivating options for increasing physical fitness are making needed contributions to the quality of late life for people who are developmentally challenged.

Retirement Adjustment

The need for planning as a prerequisite for successful adjustment to the retirement event has been acknowledged for some time by a number of advocates, planners, and professionals concerned with the well-being of older persons with mental retardation. It has been suggested (Kultgen et al., 1986; Stroud & Sutton, 1988) that persons with developmental disabilities treasure the work site because of the friendship ties developed, the money received, and the feeling of status derived from fulfilling a role that is acknowledged by the general society as normative. It is only very recently, however, that exemplary programs have been developed to teach persons with mental retardation the meaning of retirement in order to insure that they have something to retire to (Henry, 1989). Similar to their age-peers in the general society, aging persons with disabilities have been prepared for many years of productive work with little attention paid to the activity content of their retirement years. According to Cotten and Laughlin (1989):

> What is missing from educational programs for these adults is a process designed to facilitate adaptation to retirement living so that they can manage their lives at lower psychological costs and derive greater benefits from the opportunities embedded in this major transition. (p. 13)

Cotten and Laughlin (1989) describe a pre-retirement program that, although in its embryonic stage, shows promise of facilitating adjustment to retirement. This project, initiated at the Boswell Retardation Center in Sanatorium, Mississippi, yields preliminary results that show initial perceptions of life in retirement as negative. During structured interviews, participants in the project indicated their distaste by responses which showed their perception of life after employment as one with "nothing to do." When the aging persons were exposed to knowledge about part-time work, flexible schedules, and volunteer opportunities, post interviews showed more positive attitudes toward retirement.

Projects such as those undertaken at the Boswell Center need to be continued into the immediate future. The next step is to not only acquaint persons with DD to viable options to work, but to provide opportunities to learn recreational and leisure activities that are rehabilitative and habilitative. Building on established skills and past and current individual preferences is a further step.

A CALL FOR PROGRAM INNOVATIONS

The need for activities that focus on therapeutic intervention as well as involvement in normalized daily routines is evident for the population of older adults with DD. For example, opportunities to practice range of motion and joint flexibility for the purpose of slowing aging-related losses in physical reserves should be planned and interspersed within the context of normal daily activity. In other words, activities need not be removed from daily routines but rather modified to reflect a changed performance level in older adulthood; thus, addressing the original intents of programmed intervention with age sensitivity added.

The prominence of certain issues that can be directly addressed through recreative/leisure pursuits that are rehabilitative/habilitative is a direct challenge to activity professionals. These issues include physical functioning, socialization, leisure skills building for retirement, and overall health and wellness.

There is an evident need for motivating physical activities that increase or maintain gross motor function as well as enhance overall physical fitness. Social opportunities to contribute to community life, to make friends, and to feel connected to community life, can be enhanced through recreation activities that stress these components. Pre-retirement and retirement education programs that emphasize leisure awareness and skill development are urgently needed in order to smooth the transition from a work or vocational training activity focus to a retirement focus in late adulthood. Leisure opportunities that add to health, functioning, and a higher quality of life fill out the challenge list for this population. A leisure lifestyle that promotes choice and self-determination is one that recognizes the human qualities that exist in all older adults, including those with lifelong developmental challenges.

Little is known about how to appropriately assess leisure needs, interests, and skills of older adults with developmental disabilities. Matching leisure/recreative functioning information with other functional geriatric assessment data for appropriate activity program development is another area for which little clinical practice information is readily available. Activity program development and evaluation are needed in order to begin to enable both aging systems and disabilities networks, to come together to empower older adults with DD full access to community services. Programs that have been developed thus far give hope and sound evidence that older adults with DD can be successfully integrated into existing community activities and services.

REFERENCES

Allen, J. I. (1980). Jogging can modify disruptive behaviors. *Teaching Exceptional Children, 2,* 66-70.

Anderson, D. J., Lakin, K. C., Bruininks, R. H., & Hill, B. K. (1987). *A national study of residential and support services for elderly persons with mental retardation (Report No. 22).* Minneapolis, MN: University of Minnesota, Department of Educational Psychology.

Benz, M., Halpern, A., & Close, D. (1986). Access to day programs and leisure activities by nursing home residents with mental retardation. *Mental Retardation, 24*(3), 147-152.

Boyd, R., & James, A. (1990). An emerging challenge: Serving older adults with mental retardation. *Annual in Therapeutic Recreation, 1,* 56-66.

Buehler, B., Smith, B. C., & Fifield, M. G. (1985). *Medical issues in serving adults with developmental disabilities.* Logan, UT: Utah State University, Developmental Center for Handicapped Persons.

Clements, C. (1989). Quality of life project. American Association on Mental Retardation, *Aging/MR Interest Group Newsletter, 3*(3), 14.

Cotton, P. D., & Laughlin, C. S. (1989). Retirement: A new career. American Association on Mental Retardation, *Aging/MR Interest Group Newsletter, 3*(3), 13.

DiGiovanni, L. (1978). The elderly retarded: A little known group. *The Gerontologist, 18,* 262-266.

Engeman, M. W., & Pederson, E. L. (1989). Interdisciplinary health promotion program on aging adults with mental retardation. Final report submitted to the Joseph P. Kennedy Jr. Foundation. Cincinnati, OH: University Affiliated Cincinnati Center for Developmental Disorders.

Eyman, R. K., & Widaman, K. F. (1987). Life-span development of institutionalized and community-based mentally retarded persons, revisited. *American Journal of Mental Deficiency, 91,* 119-124.

Foelker, G. A., & Luke, E. A. (1989). Mental health issues for the aging mentally retarded population. *Journal of Applied Gerontology, 8*(2), 242-250.

Hawkins, B. A. (1987). Aging and developmental disability: New horizons for therapeutic recreation. *Journal of Expanding Horizons in Therapeutic Recreation, 2*(2), 42-46.

Hawkins, B. A. (1989a). Life satisfaction, activity patterns and constraints on leisure: Measurement protocols for older adults with mental retardation. In L. H. McAvoy & D. Howard (Eds.), *Abstracts for the 1989 Symposium on Leisure Research* (p. 27). Alexandria, VA: National Recreation and Park Association.

Hawkins, B. A. (1989b). Health promotion for older adults with developmental disabilities: Module 2.G. In B. A. Hawkins, S. J. Eklund, and R. P. Gaetani (Eds.), *Aging and developmental disabilities: A training inservice package.* Bloomington, IN: Indiana University Institute for the Study of Developmental Disabilities.

Hawkins, B. A., & Eklund, S. J. (1989). Aging and developmental disabilities: Interagency planning for an emerging population. *Journal of Applied Gerontology*, *8*(2), 168-174.

Hawkins, B. A., & Eklund, S. J. (1990). Planning processes and outcomes for an aging population with developmental disabilities. *Mental Retardation*, *28*(1), 35-40.

Havighurst, R. J. (1972). *Developmental tasks and education (3rd ed.)*. New York: David McKay.

Henry, N. S. (1989). Implementation of a pre-retirement training program. Paper presented at the annual meeting of the American Association on Mental Retardation, Chicago.

Jacobson, J. W., Sutton, M., & Janicki, M. P. (1985). Demography and characteristics of aging and aged mentally retarded persons. In M. P. Janicki and H. M. Wisniewski (Eds.), *Aging and developmental disabilities: Issues and approaches* (pp. 115-143). Baltimore, MD: Paul H. Brookes.

Janicki, M. P., & Jacobson, J. W. (1986). Generational trends in sensory, physical, and behavioral abilities among older mentally retarded persons. *American Journal of Mental Deficiency*, *90*, 490-500.

Janicki, M. P., & MacEachron, A. E. (1984). Residential, health and social service needs of elderly developmentally disabled persons. *The Gerontologist*, *24*, 128-137.

Janicki, M. P., Seltzer, M. M., Krauss, M. W., & Gaetani, R. P. (1989). Population overview: Module 1.A. In B. A. Hawkins, S. J. Eklund, and R. P. Gaetani (Eds.), *Aging and developmental disabilities: A training inservice package*. Bloomington, IN: Indiana University Institute for the Study of Developmental Disabilities.

Krauss, M. W. (1989). Social networks of adults with mental retardation: Reciprocity, independence, and extensiveness. Paper presented at the annual meeting of the American Association on Mental Retardation, Chicago.

Krauss, M. W., & Seltzer, M. M. (1986). Comparison of elderly and adult mentally retarded persons in community and institutional settings. *American Journal of Mental Deficiency*, *91*, 237-243.

Kultgen, P., Rinck, C., Calkins, C. F., & Intagliata, J. (1986). *Expanding the life chances and social support networks of elderly developmentally disabled adults*. Kansas City, MO: UMKC Institute for Human Development.

Lubin, R. A., & Kiely, M. (1985). Epidemiology of aging in developmental disabilities. In M. P. Janicki and H. M. Wisniewski (Eds.), *Aging and developmental disabilities: Issues and approaches* (pp. 94-114). Baltimore, MD: Paul H. Brookes.

Martz, B. L. (1989). Preventive health care: Module 2.F. In B. A. Hawkins, S. J. Eklund, and R. P. Gaetani (Eds.), *Aging and developmental disabilities: A training inservice package*. Bloomington, IN: Indiana University Institute for the Study of Developmental Disabilities.

Menolascino, F. J, & Potter, J. F. (1989). Mental illness in the elderly mentally retarded. *Journal of Applied Gerontology*, *8*(2), 192-202.

Rancourt, A. (1989). Older adults with developmental disabilities/mental retardation: Implications for professional services. *Therapeutic Recreation Journal, 23*(1), 47-57.

Rancourt, S. M. (1990). Older adults with developmental disabilities/mental retardation: A research agenda for an emerging population. *Annual in Therapeutic Recreation, 1,* 48-55.

Ray, R. O. (1990). Community leisure services: Trends and implications. Paper presented at the Outdoor Recreation Trends Symposium III, Indianapolis, IN.

Rinck, C. & Kultgen, P. (1987). Social support networks of older persons with mental retardation. Paper presented at the annual meeting of the American Association for Mental Deficiency, Los Angeles.

Rose, T. & Janicki, M. P. (1986). Older mentally retarded adults: A forgotten population. *Aging Network News, 3*(5), 17-19.

Schurrer, R., Weltman, A., & Brammell, H. (1985). Effects of physical training on cardiovascular fitness and behavior patterns of mentally retarded adults. *American Journal of Mental Deficiency, 90,* 167-169.

Seltzer, M. M. (1985). Research in social aspects of aging and developmental disabilities. In M. P. Janicki and H. M. Wisniewski (Eds.), *Aging and developmental disabilities: Issues and approaches* (pp. 161-173). Baltimore, MD: Paul H. Brookes.

Seltzer, M. M. (1989a). The impact of caregiving on aging parents with a son/daughter with mental retardation living at home. Paper presented at the annual meeting of the American Association on Mental Retardation, Chicago.

Seltzer, M. M. (1989b). Age, gender, and risk factors as predictors of aging parents' well-being. Paper presented at the annual meeting of the American Association on Mental Retardation, Chicago.

Stroud, M., & Sutton, E. (1988). *Expanding options for older adults with developmental disabilities: A practical guide to achieving community access.* Baltimore, MD: Paul H. Brookes.

Chapter 2

Developing Recreation Services to Assist Elders Who Are Developmentally Disabled

Carol Cutler Riddick
M. Jean Keller

SUMMARY. Recreation services providers should be designing and offering a continuum of recreational activities to elders with developmental disabilities (DD). A goal should be to make these individuals as independent as possible in their recreation functioning. In order to accomplish this, recreation professionals should be assisting older adults with DD acquire the knowledge and skills necessary to pursue recreational activities that are appropriate to their abilities, interests, and age level and which will foster their physical, social, mental, and/or emotional well-being. Principles and a planning process model for meeting this challenge are presented in this chapter.

OVERVIEW

Meeting the service needs of older persons with developmental disabilities (DD) has, as a topic, been neglected in the literature (Rancourt, 1989; Roberto & Nelson, 1989; Sison & Cotten, 1989).

Carol Cutler Riddick, PhD, is Associate Professor in Recreation, Gallaudet University. Requests for reprints should be sent to C. Riddick, Gallaudet University, 800 Florida Ave., N. E., Washington, DC 20002. M. Jean Keller, EdD, is Associate Professor in Recreation and Leisure Studies, University of North Texas, P.O. Box 13857, Denton, TX 76203-3857.

The authors wish to thank Sharon M. Malley, MA, CTRS, for her critical review of an earlier version of this chapter.

Although approximately 200,000 persons aged 55 years and older have one or more developmental disabilities (mental retardation, autism, cerebral palsy, or a neurological disorder), little is known on how aging affects individuals with developmental disabilities (Janicki, Knox, & Jacobson, 1985). Moreover, while evidence is available that the older population with DD is expanding, little is known how to best meet their recreation needs. Several studies have concluded that there is a lack of recreation services for individuals with disabilities (Austin et al., 1977; Lancaster, 1976; Schleien & Werder, 1985). In short, recreation services are legally mandated and some agencies and communities have accepted the responsibility of providing these services. However, principles and methods to design and implement recreation services to assist elders with DD have not been adequately developed (Schleien & Ray, 1988).

It is important to remember that elders with DD are heterogeneous in terms of their functional abilities, backgrounds, life experiences, communication abilities, social skills, and interests. Such differences, in part, explain why these individuals reside in a variety of settings including residential long term facilities, intermediate care facilities, group homes, supervised apartment complexes, foster home care, or with family members. Puccio et al. (1984) have noted the number of elders who have developmental disabilities is expected to increase in the future; while the percentage of these individuals who will reside in long term care facilities will decrease. Hence, more older adults with DD will be residing in community settings and in need of recreation services.

Given the projected increases in life expectancy experienced by persons with developmental disabilities, one major challenge confronting recreation professionals is to design and deliver recreation services that will enhance the quality of life for members of this group (Ansello & Rose, 1989). In order to assist with this undertaking, the purposes of this chapter are twofold. First, some important programming principles, to guide professionals when developing recreation services for elders with DD, will be reviewed. Second, a recreation service planning model as well as suggestions for implementing it will be proposed.

PRINCIPLES

Many recreation services professionals would agree that the following are important considerations when planning recreation programs with older persons who are developmentally disabled (Batavia, 1988; Crawford, 1986; Dattilo, 1987; McGuire & James, 1988; Rancourt, 1989; Wehman & Schleien, 1981). These principles can guide recreation professionals involved in designing appropriate recreation experiences for elders with DD.

1. *Communities should provide for a continuum of recreation services.* A series of activity options, ranging in terms from restrictive to full integration, should be offered (Taylor, 1988). Recreation services with older persons with DD should then be found in three types of settings: segregated, partially integrated, and fully integrated settings.

A segregated recreation service may be offered in an institutional or community environment. An example of a segregated service could be a craft class, offered within a group home setting, to older adults who have severe mental retardation. The rationale for offering this segregated recreation service is that these individuals may not be ready to participate in craft classes outside their group home because of their inability to read, follow complex instructions, and share materials with others. Thus, a segregated program is presented to meet these individuals' present needs and abilities.

As older adults progress towards more independent recreation functioning, partially integrated services should be made available to them. An example of partially integrated recreation service is an exercise class, designed primarily for older adults who are developmentally disabled with physical disabilities offered within a senior center setting. This exercise class would be made available to elders with non-developmental disabilities but who have physical disabilities, due to perhaps experiencing a stroke or heart attack.

When older adults with DD possess the functional abilities as well as the social skills needed to pursue recreation activities offered within the context of fully integrated settings, those activities and services are made available to them. An example of full integration would be senior adults with developmental disabilities who participate in a ceramics class offered at a community recreation center.

2. *Whenever possible, efforts should be directed to "main-stream" individuals who are disabled into generic rather than seg-regated recreation programs.* The majority of persons with disabilities prefer to be integrated into community recreation programs (Richardson et al., 1987). This principle is supported by current legislation mandates for recreation services for all individuals with disabilities and the growing numbers of older adults with DD living in communities (Schleien & Ray, 1988).

3. *In planning recreation services with elders who are developmentally disabled, professionals should abide by the least restrictive environment doctrine.* Recreation professionals should be introducing and instructing recreation skills or activities that have the potential of being performed in the presence of, or interaction with, non-disabled peers (Crawford, 1986). Also, the emphasis should be on the provision of age-appropriate recreation activities. Elders with developmental disabilities need to be exposed to recreation activities that ultimately have the potential of being pursued in partially and fully integrated settings (Crawford, 1986; Pollingue & Cobb, 1986).

4. *When planning recreation services with elders who are developmentally disabled, interagency collaboration should be sought and promoted.* Unfortunately, a major impediment to the development of service delivery to those with developmental disabilities is the lack of meaningful coordination among agencies (Sison & Cotten, 1989). Whenever possible, use of existing recreation resources should be encouraged rather than the creation of duplicating services. Recreation professionals need to develop proactive strategies to counter the common reasons for lack of interagency cooperation such as planning myopia, bureaucracy, fiscal inability, and service provider disengagement (Kenefick, 1985). For some specific ideas on how to mainstream persons with DD into existing community recreation services, see Rancourt (1989) and Richardson et al. (1987).

5. *A comprehensive recreation service planning model should be used when responding to the recreation needs of elders with devel-*

opmental disabilities. The design and delivery of recreation services are of central concern to the recreation profession; however, little information is available related to comprehensive program planning techniques and procedures to meet the recreation needs of older persons with DD. A recreation service planning model is proposed and described below.

A MODEL

A four phase model of planning recreation services for elders with developmental disabilities consists of the following steps: assessment, design, implementation, and evaluation (see Figure 1). This recreation service planning model is appropriate for all types of settings and the various functional levels of older adults with DD.

Phase 1: Assessment

The assessment phase is a multidimensional approach that requires the use of both formal and informal assessment instruments. Assessment is a systematic procedure for gathering select information about individuals for the purpose of making decisions regarding their recreation program plan (Dunn, 1984). Ideally, both the client (if their communication skills are sufficient enough to respond to posed questions) and, if appropriate, their primary caregivers should be interviewed by recreation professionals.

Three areas are being suggested for the focus of this assessment:

1. Recreation attitudes, satisfactions, preferences, abilities, and patterns, should be determined with elders who are developmentally disabled. Recreation professionals should understand the importance or value of recreation in the life of an older adult with DD and how these individuals presently spend their free time (including whether the activity is performed in integrated, partially integrated, or segregated settings). Furthermore, efforts need to be directed at determining the level of enjoyment derived from various recreation experiences. Likewise, it is important to determine leisure activities that elders have not experienced but may be interested in learning.

FIGURE 1. Recreation Services Planning Model

PHASE I - ASSESSMENT

1. Determining recreation attitudes, satisfactions, preferences, abilities, and patterns.

2. Obtaining background or profile information.

3. Discovering the availability and accessibility of community recreation resources.

PHASE II - DESIGN

1. Establishing recreation participation goals.

2. Selecting recreation options to meet goals.

3. Performing activity analysis.

PHASE III - IMPLEMENTATION

1. Considering participants.

2. Orienting and training staff.

3. Arranging and modifying facilities, equipment, and supplies.

4. Establishing the number, length, and frequency of sessions.

PHASE IV - EVALUATION

1. Determining whether or not goals were being met.

2. Establishing recreation programs and services effectiveness.

Recreational activities require various abilities and thus, individual's skills must be determined in order to create meaningful experiences. A variety of instruments exist to assess and monitor these varying aspects of recreation. For ideas on how to assess recreation behaviors and interests of persons with developmental disabilities, consult Stroud and Sutton (1988) or Wehman and Schleien (1981). For a critical evaluation of the many assessment instruments that exist to measure recreation and leisure attitudes, abilities, behaviors, satisfactions, and interests see Howe (1984). Additionally, some older adults with DD have limited response repertoires, assessment might be successfully executed and facilitated by having them interact with computers (for specifics, see Dattilo, 1988).

2. Personal background or profile information should be obtained as it can enhance or hinder recreation participation and satisfaction of older adults with DD. Background or profile data might include: what are the individual's levels of independent recreation functioning related to mental, emotional, social, and physical functioning abilities; what family or group recreational activities are these individuals excluded from because of their disability; and what financial and transportation resources are available (since these have implications for leisure activity accessibility)? It is imperative that recreation professionals working with elders with DD accept the fact that not all older adults with disabilities are capable of acquiring an independent level of recreation functioning. For ideas on how to assess independent recreation functioning, see Bates and Renzaglia, (1979:112-114).

3. The availability and accessibility of community recreation resources need to be determined. In examining accessibility, it is important to focus on the distance between community resources and elder's residence, availability of public transportation, user fees charged, and, if applicable, physical accessibility barriers (for an example of a site checklist, see Stroud & Sutton, 1988:111).

Phase 2: Design

The design phase of this model of planning recreation services to assist elders with DD insures that the assessment and implementation phases of the model are interrelated and address specific individuals' needs within the context, resources, and constraints of an agency.

1. Related to determining recreation preferences is the component of establishing recreation participation goals with elders who are developmentally disabled. Again, individuals should have input

into what they would like to accomplish through their recreational pursuits. As older persons with DD take responsibility for establishing goals for themselves, they are empowered to promote their well-being through recreation experiences and move towards more independent recreation functioning (Dattilo & Murphy, 1987). If, however, an individual's functional abilities are limited, then input should be solicited from significant others such as, family members, caregivers, or friends. If none of these options are available, then recreation professionals, after considering background information (such as functional abilities, interests, etc.) may have to surmise what goals would be appropriate, without individuals' input.

A primary consideration when designing recreation experiences is determining what do older adults with DD want, desire, or need from their leisure experiences? Recreation participation may serve many purposes for aging adults with DD—including the promotion of physical, social, mental or emotional well-being (Keller & Turner, 1986). Recreation professionals along with these older people can design appropriate recreation experiences which address the priority goals related to well-being. For instance, if it is physical well-being, then specifically does the individual want to enhance their mobility, hearing, hand coordination, speech, vision, energy level, relaxation state, etc.? If social well-being is a priority, then what is important—improving general appearance, friendliness, cooperativeness, facial expressions, relationships and interactions with others, social skills, etc.? If mental well-being emerges as an important goal for recreation activities, professionals and older adults could determine whether to promote their attention span, alertness, orientation, memory retention, ability to reason, read, write, speak, comprehension, judgement, etc. And if emotional well-being is a concern, then is it important for the person to find activities that will reduce anxiety, depression, hostility, aggressiveness, anger and/or activities designed to promote self-esteem, flexibility, feelings of usefulness etc.?

2. The intent of a goal may be accomplished through many different recreation activities. Thus, based on what is learned about elders with DD during the assessment phase, recreation professionals should determine possible recreation options to meet the goals.

The list of recreation options should be presented to older persons and their primary caregivers for consideration. Older individuals with DD should have input into the selection of their recreation activities in this phase of the planning model also.

In preparing a recreation options list with individuals, it is important to consider activities that are currently or in the past have been enjoyed by older persons with DD. Clinical experience indicates that some elders with developmental disabilities are more likely to be motivated to participate in suggested activities if these activities build on interests and skills that have been previously acquired (Janicki et al., 1985). For example, if swimming was enjoyed in youth, the older person with developmental disabilities may be open to the suggestion that they participate in a swim program.

It is also important when developing a recreation options list to consider activities that may be appealing to older individuals with DD but which they have not pursued because either they did not possess the requisite skills or had been excluded from participating with family or friends; and, that are similar to the preferences of non-disabled elders. Interestingly, favorite recreation activities and choices of older adults with developmental disabilities are typically the same as found among non-disabled elders including attending sporting events and parties, going on trips and picnics, visiting with others, going to movies, shopping, and listening to music (Stroud & Murphy, 1984).

Once a recreation options list has been prepared a planning session involving older adults, caregivers, if appropriate, and recreation professionals should be held to select recreation activity choices. Whenever possible, older people with DD should select from a list of recreation activities their choice for participation. The social psychology literature suggests that behavior change and health benefits are more likely to occur when the client is provided with an opportunity to be part of the planning process and is given the opportunity to choose a desired activity (Iso-Ahola et al., 1980; Keller & Turner, 1986).

3. Once recreation activities are selected, recreation professionals need to perform activity analyses. Activity analysis is a procedure for breaking down and examining recreation activities in terms of psychomotor, cognitive, and/or affective domains (Peterson &

Gunn, 1984). Activity analyses break down recreation activities into component behaviors, which when learned one at a time, combine to complete the mastery of recreation skills as well as empower older persons with DD to engage in meaningful recreation experiences. For an overview of how to inventory tasks see Brown et al., (1979); for sources and examples on how to conduct recreation activity analyses see Dattilo (1987) and Schleien et al. (1988:60-61); and for specific examples, see Bates and Renzaglia, (1979:117-120).

Phase 3: Implementation

Based on the information obtained during the assessment and design phases, recreation professionals will determine if, and what program adaptations or modifications should be made to create successful and meaningful recreation experiences with older adults who have developmental disabilities. Program implementation translates the assessing and designing phases into action. When recreation programs are implemented as designed, they should accomplish participants' and program's goals. During the implementation phase, recreation professionals will need to consider the participants, staff, facilities, equipment, and supplies, as well as the number, length, and frequency of recreation activity sessions (Peterson & Gunn, 1984).

1. Recreation programs should specify the intended participants, that is, for whom programs have been designed. After all, in effective recreation programming with older adults with DD, "one size does not fit all." Recreation professionals should describe abilities and prerequisite skills for programs.

Some older adults with DD who have the potential of pursuing recreation activities in partially or fully integrated settings, the implementation phase may consist of providing requisite skills to enable successful integration into community recreation programs. Primary caregivers in this instance, should be involved in assisting older persons learn and develop skills as they may be necessary to help older adults maintain these newly acquired behaviors.

Non-developmentally disabled recreation participants will need to be prepared and educated for the integration process. For instance, it has been noted that older adults are typically reluctant to accept and welcome those who are "different" into their activities. Among the reasons cited by older participants who resist interacting with their developmentally disabled counterparts are stereotypic notions about developmental disabilities, and perceptions that their image will suffer if they become involved with members of this group (Rancourt, 1989). Obviously, such concerns could become the focus of training or educational activities. All in all, previous experience suggests that integration and acceptance is a slow process and requires patience and perseverance of committed staff and volunteers (Rancourt, 1989).

Another tip for assuring success, when the goal is integration, is to establish a companion or buddy system. Older persons can be solicited to accompany other older individuals with developmental disabilities as they pursue recreational activities. These individuals can serve as role models (for social skills and behaviors) as well as become advocates for mainstreaming initiatives. Possible sources for peer companions include the Retired Senior Citizen Volunteer Program (RSVP), church groups, and associations of retired persons.

Finally, before placing older adults with DD in partially or fully integrated recreation programs, it is important to evaluate the groups and situations to determine in advance the number of persons who can be successfully placed. It could, for example, be counterproductive to place a large number of older adults with DD into a senior center since the likelihood of non-acceptance tends to increase as the numbers of persons with disabilities increase. A general rule of thumb is that mainstreaming should be done in the same proportion as disabled individuals are found in the regular population — or one disabled person for every 10 non-disabled participants (Richardson et al., 1987).

2. An additional point to consider during the implementation phases involves staff orientation and training. That is, educational efforts should be directed towards staff members in community recreation settings where integration is scheduled to take place. Inservice training typically has been helpful when it has been directed at the following topics: stereotypes about elders with developmental disabilities, awareness of the role of recreation in the lives of elders

with DD, facilitating cooperative interaction and exchange between elders with developmental disabilities and non-developmentally disabled peers, and ideas on planning recreation programs with elders' input (Dobrof, 1985; Roberto & Nelson, 1989). In short, it is important that recreation staff members possess the skills and knowledge needed to implement recreation services with persons with DD.

3. Delivering recreation services with older adults who are developmentally disabled may require modifications or adaptations to facilities, equipment, and supplies. Recreation professionals should make all necessary logistical arrangements in advance to facilitate meaningful recreation experiences.

4. The number, length, and frequency of recreation program sessions must be determined. Individual characteristics, program content, agency structure, and staffing should be considered when making decisions regarding program structure and implementation. It is also important to understand that generalization of recreation skills from learning or developmental situations to natural environments can be challenging and time consuming to achieve. This is particularly true when the skill required is beyond simple gross motor skills and environmental distractions (such as noise) are present (Crawford, 1986). The number of sessions required to achieve an objective can vary dramatically. Among the factors that influence the number of sessions offered are: abilities and learning rates of participants, task difficulty, and number of steps in activity analyses (Crawford, 1986).

Operationalizing and implementing recreation programs with older adults who are developmentally disabled can be complex. Thus, after recreation programs have been implemented, it is critical to evaluate their effectiveness so that informed decisions can be made regarding program revisions and improvements.

Phase 4: Evaluation

Evaluation has many varied meanings within the fields of developmental disabilities and recreation. Evaluation in this model is viewed as means to determine whether or not goals are being met and how to improve program or services effectiveness. As such, evaluation is an on-going process. Information is systematically gathered about the assessment, design, and implementation phases so that informed decisions about recreation programs and services can be made.

In order to determine whether or not goals are being accomplished and/or how to maximize program/service effectiveness, informal and formal data need to be collected. If the information that is collected reveals that goals are not being met or less than optimal services are being delivered, adaptation in one or more of the following areas may be warranted (Crawford, 1986):

a. Use, create, or adapt materials and devices to assist in skill acquisition during instruction.
b. Use personal assistance, such as cues, prompts, modeling, role playing, and rewards to promote achievement. Current research suggests that normal persuasion and encouragement can be one way to motivate individuals with developmental disabilities. (McGuire & James, 1988)
c. Adapt skill sequences by rearranging the order, type, number, and frequency of skills being introduced.
d. Adapt rules or revise guidelines to allow for partial participation.
e. Provide guidance or instruction to staff members, primary caregivers, and non-developmentally disabled participants to promote and enhance goal attainment.

Furthermore, when individuals have ceased participating in recreation programs, staff members should contact older adults with DD and/or primary caregivers to determine whether or not recreation experiences were satisfactory to the individuals. If the recreation experience was unsatisfactory, individual reassessment should be performed.

CONCLUSION

Recreation professionals should be designing and offering a continuum of recreational activities to elders with developmental disabilities. A goal should be to assist these individuals in their movement towards independent recreation functioning. In order to accomplish this, recreational professionals should be helping these individuals acquire the knowledge and skills necessary to pursue recreational activities that are appropriate to their abilities, interests, and age level and which will foster their physical, social, mental, and/or emotional well-being. Several principles and a recreation services planning model for meeting this challenge were presented.

The knowledge base available to the recreation profession on how to develop, maintain, and assist elders who are developmentally disabled with the expression of appropriate recreation lifestyles is limited. Hopefully, the information presented in this chapter will expand this body of knowledge as well as recreation services with older individuals who have developmental disabilities.

REFERENCES

Ansello, E.F., & Rose, T. (1989). Aging and lifelong disabilities: Problems and prospects. In E.F. Ansello & T. Rose (Eds.), *Aging and lifelong disabilities: Partnership for the twenty-first century* (pp. 9-11). Palm Springs: Elder Press.

Austin, D.R., Peterson, J.A., Peccarelli, L.M., Binkley, A., & Laker, M. (1977). *Therapeutic recreation in Indiana: Health through recreation.* Bloomington, IN: Department of Recreation and Park Administration, Indiana University.

Batavia, A. (1988). Needed: Active therapeutic recreation for high level quadriplegics. *Therapeutic Recreation Journal, 22*(2), 8-11.

Bates, P., & Renzaglia, A. (1979). Community-based recreation programs. In P. Wehman (Ed.), *Recreation programming for developmentally disabled persons* (pp. 97-126). Baltimore: University Park Press.

Brown, L., Branston, M., Hampre-Nietupski, S., Pumpian, I., Certo, N., & Grunewald, L. (1979). A strategy for developing chronologically age-appropriate and functional curricular content for severely handicapped adolescents and young adults. *The Journal of Special Education, 13*(1), 81-90.

Crawford, M. (1986). Development and generalization of lifetime leisure skills for multi-handicapped participants. *Therapeutic Recreation Journal, 20*(4), 48-60.

Dattilo, J. (1988). Assessing music preferences of persons with severe disabilities. *Therapeutic Recreation Journal, 22*(2), 12-23.

Dattilo, J. (1987). Recreation and leisure literature for individuals with mental retardation: Implications for outdoor recreation. *Therapeutic Recreation Journal, 21*(1), 9-17.

Dattilo, J., & Murphy, W. (1987). Facilitating the challenge in adventure recreation for persons with disabilities. *Therapeutic Recreation Journal, 21*(3), 14-21.

Dobrof, R. (1985). Some observations from the field of aging. In M. Janicki & H. Wisniewski (Eds.), *Aging and developmental disabilities: issues and approaches* (pp. 411-415). Baltimore, MD: Brookes Publishing Co.

Dunn, J.K. (1984). Assessment. In Peterson, C.A., & Gunn, S.L. *Therapeutic recreation program design* (pp. 267-320). Englewood Cliffs, NJ: Prentice-Hall.

Howe, C. (1984). Leisure assessment instrumentation in therapeutic recreation. *Therapeutic Recreation Journal, 18,* 17-28.

Iso-Ahola, S., MacNeil, R., & Szymanski, D. (1980). Social psychological foundations of therapeutic recreation: An attributional analysis. In S. Iso-Ahola (Ed.), *Social psychological perspectives on leisure and recreation* (pp.390-413). Springfield, IL: Charles C Thomas.

Janicki, M., Knox, L., & Jacobson, J. (1985). Planning for an older developmentally disabled population. In M. Janicki & H. Wisniewski (Eds.), *Aging and developmental disabilities: Issues and approaches* (pp. 143-160). Baltimore, MD: Brookes Publishing Co.

Keller, M., & Turner, N. (1986). Creating wellness programs with older people: A process for therapeutic recreators. *Therapeutic Recreation Journal, 20,* 6-14.

Kenefick, B. (1985). Patterns of congregate care: Existing models and future directions. In M. Janicki & H. Wisniewski (Eds.), *Aging and developmental disabilities: Issues and approaches* (pp. 351-365). Baltimore, MD: Brookes Publishing Co.

Lancaster, K. (1976). Municipal services. *Parks & Recreation, 18,* 18-27.

McGuire, F., & James, A. (1988). Attribution versus normal persuasion in the acquisition of aquatic skills by mentally retarded adults. *Therapeutic Recreation Journal, 22*(2), 24-30.

Patrick, G. (1986). The effects of wheelchair competition on self-concept and acceptance of disability in novice athletes. *Therapeutic Recreation Journal, 20*(4), 61-71.

Peterson, C.A., & Gunn, S.L. (1984). *Therapeutic recreation program design.* Englewood Cliffs, NJ: Prentice-Hall.

Pollingue, A., & Cobb, H. (1986). Leisure education: A model facilitating community integration for moderately/severely mentally retarded adults. *Therapeutic Recreation Journal, 20*(3), 54-62.

Puccio, P., Janicki, M., Otis, J., & Rettig, J. (1984). *Report of the committee on aging and developmental disabled.* Albany: Office of Mental Retardation and Developmental Disabilities.

Rancourt, A. (1989). Older adults with developmental disabilities/mental retardation: Implications for professional services. *Therapeutic Recreation Journal, 23,* 47-57.

Richardson, D., Wilson, B., Wetherald, L., & Peters, J. (1987). Mainstreaming initiative: An innovative approach to recreation and leisure services in a community setting. *Therapeutic Recreation Journal, 21*(2), 9-19.

Roberto, K., & Nelson, R. (1989). The developmentally disabled elderly: Concerns of service providers. *The Journal of Applied Gerontology, 8*, 175-182.

Schleien, S., Cameron, J., Rynders, J., & Slick, C. (1988). Acquisition and generalization of leisure skills from school to the home community by learners with severe multihandicaps. *Therapeutic Recreation Journal, 22*(3), 52-71.

Schleien, S.J., & Ray, M.T. (1988). *Community recreation and persons with disabilities*. Baltimore: Brookes Publishing Co.

Schleien, S.J., & Werder, J.K. (1985). Perceived responsibilities of special recreation services in Minnesota. *Therapeutic Recreation Journal, 19*(3), 51-62.

Sison, G., & Cotten, P. (1989). The elderly mentally retarded person: Current perspectives and future directions. *The Journal of Applied Gerontology, 8*, 151-167.

Stroud, M., & Murphy, M. (1984). *The aged mentally retarded/developmentally disabled in northeastern Ohio*. ACCESS: Cooperative Planning for Services to Aged Mentally Retarded/Developmentally Disabled Persons. (Grant to the University of Akron from the Ohio Developmental Disabilities Planning Council, No. 84-25).

Stroud, M., & Sutton, E. (1988). *Expanding options for older adults with developmental disabilities; a practical guide to achieving community access*. Baltimore, MD: Brookes Publishing Co.

Taylor, S. (1988). Caught in the continuum: Critical analysis of the principle of the least restrictive environment. *The Journal of the Association of the Severely Handicapped, 13*, 41-53.

Wehman, P. & Schleien, S. (1981). *Leisure programs for handicapped persons: Adaptations, techniques, and curriculum*. Baltimore, MD: University Park Press.

Chapter 3

Therapeutic Recreation Programming for Older Adults with Developmental Disabilities

Marcia Jean Carter
Claire Foret

SUMMARY. A growing number of aging persons with developmental disabilities are residing in the community without appropriate support services. Therapeutic recreation provides the opportunity to develop functional skills useful in the community. One approach that can be used in the development of appropriate programs is presented.

INTRODUCTION

The older adult with developmental disabilities represents a growing portion of our population. Among the large numbers of "baby boomers" entering middle age is an expanding population of adults with developmental disabilities (Sison & Cotton, 1989). The health, well-being, and life expectancy of aging adults with developmental disabilities will continue to improve as technology and concern for quality of care address their medical and social needs (Janicki, Ackerman & Jacobson, 1985; Hawkins, 1987; Rancourt, 1989).

Older adults with developmental disabilities spend a dispropor-

Marcia Jean Carter, ReD, is Associate Professor, University of Northern Iowa, E. Gym, HPER, Cedar Falls, IA 50614-0161. Claire Foret, PhD, is Assistant Professor, University of Southwestern Louisiana, Department of Health, Physical Education, and Recreation, Lafayette, LA 70506.

A grant awarded by the American Association of Leisure and Recreation, Reston, VA, facilitated this project.

35

tionate amount of time either alone, unoccupied or completing routine non-rewarding tasks (Nietupski, Hamre-Nietupski & Ayres, 1984). They find themselves excluded from "post school" habilitation programs and support resources and with limited opportunities for activity and peer interaction (Nietupski & Svoboda, 1982; Burch, Reiss & Bailey, 1985; Duffy & Nietupski, 1985). Responsibility to meet programming needs has fallen to caregivers who are outlived by the adult with developmental disabilities (Walz, Harper & Wilson, 1986; Hawkins, 1987).

Therapeutic recreation is a means for the older adult with developmental disabilities to develop and practice functional skills used in the community (Schleien, Light, McAvoy & Baldwin, 1989). The provision of therapeutic recreation services and programs is more extensive and intensive for aging adults with developmental disabilities than for other age groups with only one disability. The older adult with developmental disabilities has experienced severe, chronic physical and/or mental impairments since childhood in three or more areas: self-care, receptive and expressive language, learning, mobility, self-direction, independent living, and economic sufficiency (Carter, VanAndel & Robb, 1985). The development of functional skills must be individually planned and coordinated by trained professionals throughout the life of the aging adult with developmental disabilities (Burch, Reiss & Bailey, 1985).

The purpose of this chapter is to present one approach in designing therapeutic recreation programs for older adults with developmental disabilities. In the model (see Figure 1), the therapeutic recreation process is adapted to incorporate task analytic leisure skill training and observation assessment methods found successful with adults with severe disabilities (Dattilo, 1984; Nietupski, Hamre-Nietupski & Ayres, 1984). The approach is designed as a training model to facilitate coordination among caregivers and professionals as activity plans are developed for aging adults with developmental disabilities.

STEP 1: ASSESS BEHAVIORS

Assessment is the process of gathering information to make appropriate activity selections. The first area assessed is the ability of the older adult with developmental disabilities to perform the re-

FIGURE 1. Therapeutic Recreation Programming for Older Adults with Developmental Disabilities

Step 1 ASSESS BEHAVIORS

    Record behaviors during leisure experiences

    Observe leadership intervention required

    Document environmental influences

Step 2 ACTIVITY SELECTION

    Determine activity preferences

    Determine compatibility of leadership and environmental

        factors to activity preferences

Step 3 DEVELOP INDIVIDUALIZED PROGRAM

    Write performance objectives and establish performance

        criteria

    Write task sequences

    Identify adaptation and modification strategies

    Select lead-up and follow-up activities

FIGURE 1 (continued)

Step 4 MONITOR AND EVALUATE EXPERIENCES

Monitor leadership interventions

Record responses

Analyze environmental influences

Step 5 FOLLOW-UP

Adjust performance objectives and criteria

Adjust task sequences

Adjust leadership interventions

Review environmental factors

Recommend prerequisite skills or lead-up activities

Implement follow-up or maintenance and generalization
activities

quirements of an activity. Secondly, the amount of leadership given to the older adult with developmental disabilities is determined. Lastly, the environmental factors influencing the adult's participation in the activities are recorded. Observation of adults as they participate in task analyzed activities has been identified as an appropriate assessment method for adults with developmental disabilities (Dattilo, 1984). An activity that has been task analyzed is one in which the skills are broken down or listed in sequential steps from the first to the last skill to be demonstrated during the activity. The task analysis of horseshoes is illustrated in Figure 2. Each skill in the sequence may be observed to determine the ability of the older adult to perform the activity. Persons trained as observers record the correctness with which the skills are displayed over several observation periods.

The second area assessed is the amount of assistance given to the older adult with development disabilities by the leader. Five levels of assistance are operationally defined and given numerical codes (see Figure 3): (1) full assistance; (2) partial assistance; (3) modeling; (4) gestural; and (5) independent. The trained observer records the number of the level which best represents the amount of assistance given by the leader.

The third area assessed is the factors within the activity setting that influence participation by the older adult with developmental disabilities. These factors are adjusted by the leader to recognize the adult's preferences and abilities. Information is recorded on the group size and the adult to leader ratio, the type of activity setting, the physical position of the adult, the assistance given to the adult, and the types of reinforcers and precautions used during the activity.

STEP 2: ACTIVITY SELECTION

The selection of activities to use during the unobligated time of an older adult with development disabilities is influenced by the information gathered during the assessment process and by the preferences shown during activity participation. Adults are observed as they participate in a variety of potential activities. Those activities that are completed correctly over several observation periods and for which the time of participation remains the same and/or in-

FIGURE 2. Task Analysis of Horseshoes

Objective with narrative: To release and retrieve horseshoes to and from stake a distance of 5-20 feet. Toss horseshoes so they land near or on stake. Underhand motion is recommended. Tasks may be completed from either standing or seated position. Horseshoes are to be held in dominate hand.

Prerequisite Skills: Palmar grasp and release, visual tracking, swing arm forward and backward

Material: Horseshoe set

Task Steps   Leadership Levels

1. Underhand grasp of   1. Full assistance, leader's hand over
   horseshoe   adult's hand, verbal cue, pick up
                                  the horseshoe.

                              2. Partial assistance, leader's hand on
                                  adult's wrist, verbal cue, pick up the
                                  horseshoe.

                              3. Modeling, leader demonstrates complete
                                  task and requests adult to complete as
                                  shown.

                              4. Gestural, leader points to horseshoe,
                                  verbal cue, pick up horseshoe.

                              5. Independent, leader places equipment
                                  before adult, states adult's name, and
                                  requests adult to grasp object.

2. Hold horseshoe and swing arm backward

1. Hand over adult's hand holding horseshoe, verbal cue, hold horseshoe and swing your arm back and forth.
2. Hand on adult's wrist, verbal cue, hold object and swing your arm back and forth.
3. Leader demonstrates complete task and requests adult to complete as shown.
4. Point to adult's hand, verbal cue, hold object and swing your arm back and forth.
5. State adult's name, and request that adult hold object.

3. Release horseshoe so it lands in target area

1. Hand over adult's hand, verbal cue, release the object toward the target.
2. Hand on adult's wrist, verbal cue, release the object toward the target.
3. Leader demonstrates complete task and requests adult to complete as shown.
4. Point to hand held object then to target, verbal cue, release the object to the target.
5. State adult's name, and request adult to release object.

FIGURE 2 (continued)

4. Repeat task steps 1-3 for toss of each horseshoe.

5. Pick up horseshoes

Repeat five steps with each target throw.

1. Leader moves to target area with hand on adult's hand, verbal cue, pick up and hold objects for next throw.

2. Leader moves to target area, with hand at adult's wrist, verbal cue, pick-up and held objects for next throw.

3. Leader demonstrates complete task and requests adult to complete as shown.

4. Leader moves to target area, points to adult's hand and objects, verbal cue, pick up objects.

5. State adult's name and request that adult pick-up objects.

FIGURE 3. Leadership Intervention

Leader uses verbal, physical and or gestural cues to
communicate to adult how to perform the skill. The five levels
represent a cue hierarchy with the leader giving the adult the
most assistance at level 1, full assistance, and the least
assistance at level 5, independent.

1. Full assistance

Direct the adult's attention to the skill. Assist the adult
through complete skill by physically manipulating the adult's
limbs. Throughout skill completion verbally cue the adult to
complete each step in the skill with the leader.

2. Partial Assistance

Direct adult's attention to the skill. Manually assist
the adult during each step in the skill as needed and until the
skill is completed. Verbally cue the adult throughout skill
completion.

FIGURE 3 (continued)

3. Modeling

Direct the adult's attention to the skill. Demonstrate how to perform skill. Indicate to adult to do just what the leader does to complete the skill. Verbally cue the adult throughout skill completion.

4. Gestural

Direct the adult's attention to the skill. Point to equipment or activity resources and adult and verbally cue the adult to complete skill.

5. Independent

Give adult verbal cue to initiate and complete skill.

creases with each observation are potential choices of the older adult with developmental disabilities. Selection of activities is determined by the compatibility of the adult's skills and preferences with the leadership and support resources available to offer the activity. Thus, leaders need to have alternative activities available to accommodate the choices made by the older adult with developmental disabilities.

STEP 3: INDIVIDUALIZED PROGRAM

Information from assessing and observing the older adult's activity preferences are considered as the activity plan is designed. The first step in the development of individualized program plans is the writing of performance objective statements. These statements specify the behaviors to be completed and the criteria to determine the success of the older adult's performance. They identify the skills for which task sequences are written. Also, performance objective statements establish the criterion used in the evaluation and monitoring process.

The second step in the development of the individualized program plan is the analyses of the behaviors in the performance objective statements to determine the sequence of skills necessary to complete each activity. These skills are listed in a task sequence and are numbered beginning with the first, assigned the number one (1), continuing to the last step, assigned the highest numerical value.

After writing performance objectives and preparing task sequences, adaptations are identified. Leadership techniques, skills, and procedures governing the activity are adapted to accommodate the multiple needs of the older adult with developmental disabilities. First, the leader selects one of the five levels of assistance to present an activity. If the older adult is unable to successfully demonstrate the skill at, for example, partial assistance, the leader introduces additional help and presents the activity at the level of full assistance.

Second, adaptation of the skills in a task sequence occurs when the leader selects the skill level at which participation will begin. If the older adult with developmental disabilities completes the skill level chosen by the leader, the next steps in the task sequence are attempted. The leader moves back to the previous step in the sequence when difficulty occurs.

Third, the activity procedures are adapted to eliminate any participation barriers for the older adult with developmental disabilities. Redesigning equipment, rule modification, and altering the number of attempts exemplify procedural adaptations. For example, if five tosses of the horseshoes rather than three results in more success this becomes an appropriate adaptation.

The last step in the development of individualized program plans is the selection of lead-up and follow-up activities. These activities are introduced prior to and after presenting a particular task sequence to enhance the use of a skill by the older adult with developmental disabilities in the current and future settings. These activities may be adaptations of the original activity or alternative ways to display the skills in an activity. A lead-up or prerequisite activity to horseshoes might be to drop or to throw the horseshoes into targets such as boxes. A follow-up activity to horseshoes might be other target games such as ring toss or lawn darts.

STEP 4: MONITOR AND EVALUATE PARTICIPANT EXPERIENCES

Monitoring and evaluation occur as the older adult with developmental disabilities is observed during recreation activities. Documentation enables leaders and caregivers to share information so consistency during program delivery is encouraged. Information is recorded on the observation form (see Figure 4) by either the activity leader or an observer of the activity who records information independent of the leader.

Columns on the observation form permit entry of the following information: The date on which the observation occurs; the numerical value of the skill or entry level task in which the older adult with developmental disabilities is recreating; the numerical value of the leadership assistance (1 through 5); the correctness (correct +, incorrect −) and the time of participation; and, the response rate. The remainder of the form permits the observer to enter anecdotal notes on the environmental factors in the setting.

The following case study is presented to illustrate the use of the

FIGURE 4. Observation Form

Client: ___David___

Objective: To release and retrieve the
___horseshoes to and from the stake___   Criterion for success: ___70%___

Trials
Response Correct+, Incorrect-
by Time, seconds

Date	Entry Level Task	Leadership Intervention Level	1	2	3	4	5	6	7	8	9	10	Response Rate%
1990	3	3	+/5	-/0	+/5	-/0	+/5	+/6	+/7	+/7	+/7	+/7	80

FIGURE 4 (continued)

Environmental Contingencies:

Group Size (staff-client ratio):

(1-1) _____ dual _X_ small group (3-4) _____ large group (4+) _____

Physical Setting: Segregated _____
Integrated within residence or social placement _X_
Integrated in community placement _____

Client Position: Prone _____ Supine _____ Sitting (w/c) _X_ Standing _____

Client Assistance: Unassisted _____
Assisted by person _X_
Assisted by apparatus _____
Assisted by person and apparatus _____

Client Reinforcers: _____Congratulatory handshakes_____

Client Precautions: _____Tends to lean forward to maintain balance_____ observation form to monitor and evaluate an older adult with developmental disabilities who is participating in horseshoes. David's objective is to release and retrieve the horseshoes to and from the stake with a success rate of 70%. This information is recorded on the proper lines. The date of the observation is recorded in the column under the proper heading. David grasps and holds the horseshoes so the leader begins instruction at step 3, release of the horseshoes to the stake. This number is recorded under the column "Entry Level Task." David complies when shown how to complete a skill. Therefore, modeling is the leadership level (number 3) chosen to present the skill. Number "3" is entered under the heading "Leadership Intervention Level." David correctly (+) releases the horseshoes to the stake eight (8) of the 10 observations. Thus, David's response rate is 80% which is above his criterion of 70%. The recorded time in seconds identifies whether the activity is sustained. David's response time consistently increased. From the collected data, the leader determines that horseshoes is a potential recreation activity to use during David's unobligated time.

The conditions present as David recreated are noted under "Environmental Contingencies." David participated with his roommate (dual) in the activity room (integrated within residence) sitting in his wheelchair assisted by the leader. The leader reinforced David's behavior with congratulatory handshakes. David experiences difficulty balancing in his wheelchair. The leader notes his tendency to lean forward under the heading "Client Precautions."

STEP 5: FOLLOW-UP

During the final phase of programming, the individual plan is reviewed to determine if adjustments are needed in the performance objectives and criteria, task sequences, leadership techniques, and environmental contingencies. Also, the leader makes recommendations on appropriate leisure activities and environmental factors. In David's case, the criterion for success may be increased from 70% to 80% or higher. David's skill level would also suggest that he might enjoy such follow-up target games as lawn darts or ring toss. David may also be able to develop a skill with less leadership assistance so a leader might be able to use gestural assistance. Also because David was successful with his roommate within his residence, the next step might be to participate with three or four other older adults with developmental disabilities at a park in the community.

CONCLUSION

The use of this process creates a data base to justify selection of recreation experiences for older adults with developmental disabilities with multiple needs. The programming process is individualized and documented so caregivers and professionals may coordinate their efforts. Through therapeutic recreation experiences, the growing number of older adults with developmental disabilities entering and remaining in the community may acquire functional skills which enable use of unobligated time and enhance community living.

REFERENCES

Burch, M. R., Reiss, M., & Bailey, J. S. (1985). A facility-wide approach to recreation programming for adults who are severely and profoundly retarded. *Therapeutic Recreation Journal, XIX*(3), 71-78.

Carter, M. J., VanAndel, G. E., & Robb, G. M. (1985). *Therapeutic recreation, a practical approach.* St. Louis: Times Mirror/Mosby College Publishing.

Dattilo, J. (1984). Therapeutic recreation assessment for individuals with severe handicaps. In G. Hitzhusen (Ed.), *Expanding Horizons in Therapeutic Recreation XI* (pp. 147-157). Columbia: University of Missouri.

Duffy, A. T., & Nietupski, J. (1985). Acquisition and maintenance of video game initiation, sustaining and termination skills. *Education and Training of the Mentally Retarded, 20* (2), 157-162.

Hawkins, B. (1987). Aging and developmental disability; new horizons for therapeutic recreation. *Journal of Expanding Horizons in Therapeutic Recreation, 2* (2), 42-46.

Nietupski, J. A., Hamre-Nietupski, S., & Ayres, B. (1984). Review of task analytic leisure skill training efforts: practitioner implications and future research needs. *Journal of the Association for the Severely Handicapped, 9* (2), 88-97.

Nietupski, J., & Svoboda, R. (1982). Teaching a cooperative leisure skill to severely handicapped adults. *Education and Training of the Mentally Retarded, 17* (1), 38-43.

Rancourt, A. M. (1989). Older adults with developmental disabilities/mental retardation: implications for professional services. *Therapeutic Recreation Journal, 23* (1), 47-57.

Schleien, S. J., Light, C. L., McAvoy, L. M., & Baldwin, C. K. (1989). Best professional practices: serving persons with severe multiple disabilities. *Therapeutic Recreation Journal, 23* (3), 27-40.

Singh, N. N., & Millichamp, C. J. (1987). Independent and social play among profoundly mentally retarded adults: training, maintenance, generalization, and long-term follow-up. *Journal of Applied Behavior Analysis, 20* (1), 23-34.

Sison, G. F. P., & Cotten, P. D., (1989). The elderly mentally retarded person: current perspectives and future directions. *The Journal of Applied Gerontology, 8* (2), 151-167.

Walz, T., Harper, D., & Wilson, J. (1986). The aging developmentally disabled person: a review. *The Gerontologist, 26* (6), 622-629.

Chapter 4

Using Needs Assessment to Develop Programs for Elderly Developmentally Disabled Persons in a Rural Setting

Claudia J. See
David N. Ellis
Charles R. Spellman
Pamela J. Cress

SUMMARY. The Needs Assessment for Adults with Developmental Disabilities (NAADD) was developed and field tested on 60 aging adults with developmental disabilities. This instrument is described and selected results of the field test are reported. The ways in which these results were used for program planning are reported. Recommendations are made for planning programs to provide community-based services for elderly persons with developmental disabilities based on needs assessments and utilization of community resources.

Until recently, little attention was given to aging persons who experience developmental disabilities. Now, national attention is being focused on the special needs of this group and their right to services (Janicki & Wisniewski, 1985; Gambert, Liesbeskind, &

Claudia J. See is with Class LTD, P.O. Box 266, Columbus, KS 66725. David N. Ellis, Charles R. Spellman and Pamela J. Cress are affiliated with the University of Kansas, Bureau of Child Research.

The authors wish to acknowledge the support of the Kansas Department on Aging and Class LTD, Columbus, KS.

Cameron, 1987; Herrera, 1983). It has been predicted that the number of individuals in the United States over the age of 55 will increase 39% by the year 2000 and 87% before 2020 (Janicki & Wisniewski, 1985). Assuming that the number of aging persons with developmental disabilities increases at a similar rate, there will be a severe shortage of service options for elderly persons with developmental disabilities. Persons with developmental disabilities who are now middle-aged or older have not had the opportunity to live, work, and/or play in integrated environments. They have lived in institutions, nursing homes, group homes, and other settings which limit personal experiences with community health, social, and recreational resources. It has been and may continue to be the responsibility of service provision agencies to assist their clientele in the full utilization of these resources.

Providing comprehensive services for this population requires a knowledge of the needs of potential consumers. While the problems faced by agencies which serve rural areas are comparable with those in urban areas, factors such as low incidence, great distances, and life style diversity make service provision problematic. In order to gain information about the needs of elderly persons with developmental disabilities living in a rural area, a survey instrument, the Needs Assessment for Adults with Developmental Disabilities (NAADD), was designed. The purpose of this chapter is to report on the field test of the NAADD and to detail how the results of the survey were used in program planning both agency-wide and for individual clients.

SURVEY INSTRUMENT

The NAADD uses an interview format to obtain information from the client or an informant who is familiar with the client. It is divided into the following sections: *General Information, Physical and Health Conditions, Nutritional Information, Maladaptive Behaviors, Service Needs,* and *Leisure and Recreation Preferences.* The *General Information* provides information about the individual's residential history, current living arrangements and some personal characteristics. The *Physical and Health Conditions* details the current physiological status of the subject. The *Nutritional In-*

formation section provides a brief summary of eating habits and overall nutritional status. The frequency and severity of aggressive and other socially inappropriate behavior is obtained from the *Maladaptive Behaviors* section. The *Service Needs* section ascertains areas where additional services are needed and the priority level of the need. The *Leisure and Recreation Preferences* section questions the respondent about desired activities.

The survey was field tested and revised after use with 60 elderly persons with developmental disabilities. The survey instrument is included and may be reproduced without the permission of the authors (see Figure 1).

FIELD TEST

Respondents

The search for subjects was conducted through presentations to civic groups, newspaper advertisements, and service agencies. A population of 90 persons with developmental disabilities who were 45 years of age or older was identified.

Persons considered developmentally disabled have physical or mental impairments whose onset was prior to 22 years of age and that result in significant dysfunction in self-care, language, learning, mobility, self-direction, independent living, or economic self-sufficiency. These persons typically require a combination and sequence of special, interdisciplinary, or generic care, treatment, or other services which are of lifelong or extended duration and are individually planned and coordinated (Federal Developmental Disabilities Act).

Not all the individuals located were surveyed. Permission was obtained to interview 60 persons. These persons lived in rural southeast Kansas and ranged in age from 45 to 73 years with 33 males and 27 females, respectively. Respondents were the individual, his or her parents, employees of service provision agencies, or other caregivers. All interviews were conducted by the senior author.

FIGURE 1

NEEDS ASSESSMENT FOR ADULTS WITH DEVELOPMENTAL DISABILITIES
(NAADD)

Name _____ DOB_____

Site Address _____ Phone_____

Contact Person_____ Phone_____

Section 1: GENERAL INFORMATION

Sex   M   F   MR level_____ Adaptive behavior level _____

RESIDENCE

Own family ___ Group home ___ Indep___ Nursing home___ Other___

Residential History _____

Dates _____ Location_____

Dates _____ Location_____

Dates _____ Location_____

Originating county _____

Position in household_____

Number in household _____ Sources of income _____

Monthly income _____

Religious preference _____

Guardian _____

Guardian _____

Data collector _____

SOURCES OF INFORMATION:

Interview with subject_____Individual habilitation plan _____

Caregiver interview _____Staff of residential facility_____

Case manager _____Family member_____

Section 2: HEALTH AND PHYSIOLOGICAL STATUS

Do you have a problem with:

General health   YES NO

When was the last time you visited your doctor?_____

What was the purpose of the visit? _____

_____

Vision   YES NO

When was the last time you visited your eye doctor?_____

What was the reason for the visit? _____

_____

Hearing   YES NO

When was the last time you had your hearing tested? _____

What was the reason for the visit_____

_____

Teeth or Gums   YES NO

When was the last time you visited your dentist?_____

What was the reason for the visit_____

_____

Limbs   YES NO

Describe the problems you have with your arms and/or legs_____

_____

Joints   YES NO

Describe the problems you have with your joints_____

_____

Ambulation   YES NO

What problems do you encounter in trying to move around_____

_____

CHRONIC CONDITIONS   MEDICATION AND SCHEDULE

___ Heart disease   _____

___ Circulatory   _____

FIGURE 1 (continued)

___ Seizures

___ Diabetes

___ Parkinson

___ Cerebral Palsy

___ Cancer

___ Ulcer

___ Tardive Dyskinesia

___ Other _____

Section 3: NUTRITIONAL INFORMATION

Weight _____   Height _____

Underweight_____   Normal_____   Overweight_____   Obese_____

Special diet _____

Food texture _____

Do you eat? Breakfast AM Snack   Lunch   PM Snack   Bedtime Snack

Who fixes the meals?_____

Favorite food _____

When was the last time you had that?_____

Do you eat out? _____ Where? _____

Section 4: MALADAPTIVE BEHAVIORS

	Frequency	Severity low high
Verbal aggression	H D W M	1 2 3 4 5 6 7
Physical aggression	H D W M	1 2 3 4 5 6 7
Nonparticipation	H D W M	1 2 3 4 5 6 7

Socially inappropriate	H	D	W	M		1 2 3 4 5 6 7
Self-injurious		H	D	W	M	1 2 3 4 5 6 7
Withdrawn		H	D	W	M	1 2 3 4 5 6 7
Stealing		H	D	W	M	1 2 3 4 5 6 7
Property destruction	H	D	W	M		1 2 3 4 5 6 7
Fearful, anxious		H	D	W	M	1 2 3 4 5 6 7
Depressed		H	D	W	M	1 2 3 4 5 6 7
Wanders		H	D	W	M	1 2 3 4 5 6 7

Behavior programs_____

H=hourly; D=daily; W=weekly; M=monthly

Section 5: SERVICE NEEDS

What do you think are some of the areas of your life where some needs
are not being met? _____

_____

Do you need help in the area of:

Area		Priority of need	
		low high	
Mental Health	YES NO	1 2 3 4 5 6 7	_____
Dental Services	YES NO	1 2 3 4 5 6 7	_____
Area		**Priority of need**	
		low high	
Health Care	YES NO	1 2 3 4 5 6 7	_____
Vision	YES NO	1 2 3 4 5 6 7	_____
Hearing	YES NO	1 2 3 4 5 6 7	_____
Medical Equipment	YES NO	1 2 3 4 5 6 7	_____
Speech	YES NO	1 2 3 4 5 6 7	_____
Transportation			
To Town	YES NO	1 2 3 4 5 6 7	_____

FIGURE 1 (continued)

Around Town	YES NO	1 2 3 4 5 6 7	_____
Between Towns	YES NO	1 2 3 4 5 6 7	_____
Work	YES NO	1 2 3 4 5 6 7	_____
Rehabilitation	YES NO	1 2 3 4 5 6 7	_____
Residential	YES NO	1 2 3 4 5 6 7	_____
Meals	YES NO	1 2 3 4 5 6 7	_____
Homemaking	YES NO	1 2 3 4 5 6 7	_____
Home Safety	YES NO	1 2 3 4 5 6 7	_____
Advocacy/Guardian	YES NO	1 2 3 4 5 6 7	_____
Legal	YES NO	1 2 3 4 5 6 7	_____
Recreation/Leisure	YES NO	1 2 3 4 5 6 7	_____
Exercise/Fitness	YES NO	1 2 3 4 5 6 7	_____
Senior Friends	YES NO	1 2 3 4 5 6 7	_____
Adult Day Care	YES NO	1 2 3 4 5 6 7	_____

Other areas_____

_____

Additional Comments _____

_____

Section 6: Leisure and Recreational Preferences

What are some activities you enjoy doing for free time?_____

_____

What are some activities that you feel you might enjoy doing?_____

_____

_____

Do you like to: Comments

Watch. Television   YES NO   _____

Play table games	YES	NO
Play active games	YES	NO
Exercise/walk	YES	NO
Garden/house plants	YES	NO
Household chores	YES	NO
Needlework	YES	NO
Paint	YES	NO
Woodwork/leatherwork	YES	NO
Crafts	YES	NO
Listen to music	YES	NO
Read	YES	NO
Photography	YES	NO
Have a pet	YES	NO
Fish	YES	NO
Camp	YES	NO
Shop	YES	NO
Sing	YES	NO
Dance	YES	NO
Swim	YES	NO
Bowl	YES	NO
Cook	YES	NO
Play cards	YES	NO
Watch sports	YES	NO
Play sports	YES	NO
Go to movies	YES	NO
Lectures	YES	NO
Eating out	YES	NO

FIGURE 1 (continued)

Traveling	YES NO	_____
Senior center	YES NO	_____
Special interests	YES NO	_____
Pen pal/write letters	YES NO	_____

Results

The results from the Service Needs section of the survey are summarized in Table 1. This table corresponds to items and responses found in the Service Needs section of the NAADD survey instrument. This section of the instrument identifies areas in which services may be needed and rates the priority of these needs using a Likert-type scale (1 = low priority; 7 = high priority).

Transportation for traveling between towns was reported as needed by the largest percentage of respondents (80%). Thirty-eight percent of these persons considered this a high priority (scores of 5 to 7 on the Likert-type scale).

Seventy-two percent of the respondents indicated that they needed assistance in obtaining employment. However, this was not considered a high priority by these persons.

A number of the respondents indicated that they needed assistance in obtaining services in the area of senior friends (35%), exercise/fitness (30%), recreation (30%), and hearing services (29%). Although these percentages fall in the middle of the distribution of areas of need, they represent high priorities to those in need. Less than 20% of the respondents indicated that they needed assistance in the areas of dental services, vision, and health care. The remaining 13 categories were needed by 5% or less of the respondents. It is important to note, though, that many of these areas that were needed by few respondents were a high priority, for example, transportation to town, legal, mental health, medical equipment, and adult day care.

<u>Table 1</u>. The percent of those surveyed who reported they needed help in each area and the percent of those among them who felt that it was a high priority area (scores of 5 to 7 on the Likert-type scale).

Need Area	Needing Help %	High Priority %
Mental Health	1	100
Dental Services	17	35
Health Care	10	30
Vision	10	20
Hearing	29	69
Medical Equipment	1	100
Speech	5	0
Work	72	18
Rehabilitation	5	0
Residential/Leisure	0	0
Meals	0	0
Homemaking	0	0
Home Safety	1	0
Advocacy/Guardian	0	0
Legal	3	67
Recreation	30	53
Exercise/Fitness	30	63
Senior Friends	35	63
Adult Day Care	1	100
<u>Transportation:</u>		
To Town	3	67
Around Town	5	40
Between Towns	80	38

Utilization of the Field Test

The survey indicated the need for opportunities to interact with peers in a social environment. An informal survey determined that there were few existing community options which could fill this need. To address this need a program was created which provided elderly developmentally disabled persons with group recreational and leisure activities. Although many of the activities offered by this program are community-based, it remains segregated. The agency continues to place a high priority on the use of integrated community-based programs to meet the recreational and leisure needs of these persons.

Several persons who were surveyed using the NAADD have begun to access existing services in their communities. The identification of individual needs using the assessment tool enabled the support staff to locate appropriate services.

Case studies will follow to highlight ways of providing community-based services for elderly persons with DD. The program planning process is based on individual needs assessments and utilization of community resources.

Case Study 1

Harry was a 63-year-old retiree living in a senior citizen housing complex. The NAADD showed that Harry was in need of a hearing aid and part-time employment. Harry was referred to an audiologist who prescribed a hearing aid. However, due to lack of personal funds Harry was unable to purchase a hearing device. Harry was then referred to an organization that helps persons obtain hearing devices. Through the help of a job coach a part-time position was located in a factory and training was provided until Harry was capable of performing the task.

Case Study 2

Sally was 59 years of age and lived with her daughter. Needs were identified in the areas of transportation, work, living facilities, legal, recreation, exercise, senior friends, health care and vision. Her need in the area of vision remains unresolved. Further evaluation is necessary to determine whether she needs a change in her lens prescription. To date, funding for this medical service has not been obtained. Sally was referred to several service providers who have helped her address most of her other identified needs through the following services:

1. low cost senior citizen transportation system,
2. an apartment in a senior citizen housing complex,
3. advice from legal aid,
4. a senior center which provides recreation, senior friends, and health screenings,
5. exercise classes at the YMCA.

Case Study 3

April was 58 years of age and lived in the family home by herself. Her income was derived from the sale of cosmetics and homemade crafts in her community. April's needs were in the areas of health care and employment. Her extremely small community offered limited work opportunities and there was no public transportation. Green Thumb, a federally funded program that was accessed through the Area Agency on Aging, found employment for April as a lunch aide at the local high school. Health care needs were met through referral to a local physician.

CONCLUSION AND RECOMMENDATIONS

When older persons with developmental disabilities live together in institutions or in other communal facilities it is possible for social agencies to adopt a one-size-fits-all approach to service provision. Using this approach many of the service needs addressed by the NAADD are filled by agency employees. However, when agencies seek to serve older persons with developmental disabilities in large rural areas where people live and work in a variety of environments, meeting the needs of these persons becomes problematic. The NAADD is an efficient means for monitoring the ongoing needs of aging persons with developmental disabilities in such settings.

As needs for services for persons with developmental disabilities are identified, agencies and individuals interested in this population often meet these needs by designing "special" programs. These programs typically exclude persons without disabilities. Special Olympics, special education, group homes, institutions, and sheltered workshops are examples of programs that have been created for persons with disabilities. What is considered "best practice" today is to provide integrated, rather than segregated services (Janicki & Wisniewski, 1985). When new service needs are identified for persons with developmental disabilities the creation of "special" services is to be avoided. Older adults with developmental disabilities should be integrated into existing services, with additional training and support as needed. When services are not available, new services should be designed for and used by all older persons who could benefit.

REFERENCES

Gambert, S.R., Liebeskind, S., & Cameron, D. (1987). Lifelong preventative health care for elderly persons with disabilities. *Journal of Association for Persons with Severe Handicaps*, *12*, 292-296.

Herrera, P.M. (1983). *Innovative programming for the aging and aged*. Exploration Series Press: Akron, Ohio.

Janicki, M.P., & Wisniewski, H.M. (1985). *Aging and developmental disabilities: Issues and approaches*. Baltimore: Paul H. Brookes.

Stokes, T.F., & Baer, D.M. (1977). An implicit technology of generalization. *Journal of Applied Behavior Analysis*, *10*, 349-367.

Chapter 5

The Use of Art Therapy for Older Adults with Developmental Disabilities

Jane E. Harlan

SUMMARY. A model program is described for elders with mental retardation, based upon the concept of art as therapy. Its goals are to provide (1) an age-appropriate creative activity for a population which often lacks meaningful retirement pursuits; (2) exploration of the developmental issues of aging; and (3) creative expression fostering an increase in self-esteem and autonomous functioning. Topics include the role of the art therapist, motivation of participants, responding to the art work, and promoting autonomy. The impact of the art experience on the participants and implications for future program development are also discussed.

INTRODUCTION

"What do I have to show for my life?" This question was asked by a 59-year-old woman who regrets never having had the opportunities for accomplishment provided by education, employment, marriage and parenthood. She articulates a dilemma faced by many older persons with mental retardation. Early in life, she and others of her generation were isolated from family and community within institutions. Persons with developmental disabilities are now entering their later years with unfulfilled potential and an inadequate repetoire of meaningful retirement activities. They are also faced

Jane E. Harlan has a master's degree in art therapy from New York University, and is currently Research Associate at Indiana University.

The author acknowledges the support of the Program on Aging at the Institute for the Study of Developmental Disabilities.

67

with developmental tasks associated with aging, such as adaptation to losses and physical changes, which they may be ill-equipped to negotiate due to cognitive limitations, emotional difficulties, and/or environmental deprivation.

Based upon the response of participants in a recently established model art therapy program, it appears that creative art experiences are well suited to fulfill the dual purpose of providing much needed activity skills and addressing the age-specific concerns of this newly emerging population. Areas of functioning which are positively impacted include self-esteem, span of attention, and productive expression of mourning over loss, anger and other feelings.

The program described here uses the concept of *art as therapy*. Art therapy as a treatment modality for a wide range of populations has been described by major theoretician-practitioners such as Margaret Naumburg (1973), Edith Kramer (1971), and Judith Rubin (1984). The "art as therapy" approach exploits a healing potential inherent in the creative process. The task of putting an image, seen or imagined, onto paper or into clay causes our inner experience to be more accessible to ourselves and to others. Integrating aspects of our cognitive abilities, emotional make-up, and life experience, the resulting art work is uniquely ours. It is tangible and can be shared with and acknowledged by those around us.

There is an absence of literature on the use of art therapy with older persons with mental retardation. This modality has been used extensively with non-developmentally disabled older persons in nursing homes, hospitals and day programs (Jungels, 1982; Rugh, 1985; Weiss, 1984, and others). The focus of such work has been on building self-esteem and a sense of dignity, strengthening cognitive skills, reminiscence, and other issues of aging. Art therapists have also described their work with younger adults with mental retardation (Kunkle-Miller, 1978; O'Malley, 1978; Wilson, 1977). Many gains in areas such as autonomous functioning, fine motor coordination and elimination of self-abusive behavior reflect the impact of the art experience for that population.

The necessity of designing quality day programing for the special needs of seniors with developmental disabilities has only recently begun to be recognized. There is also a shortage of activity professionals and therapists trained in the fields of aging and mental retardation available to create such programing. Within this context, the

Institute for the Study of Developmental Disabilities at Indiana University has initiated a pilot art therapy program at a group home in the southeastern part of the state. Residents are persons with mental retardation, ranging in age from 57 to 71. Seven out of eight of the residents have participated in an art group held once a week for an hour and a half, over a period of 7 months. The program has been designed and implemented by the author.

The program goals are to provide a model for (1) an age-appropriate, creative activity for older persons with developmental disabilities; (2) an avenue for exploration of age-specific issues such as reminiscence, decline of health status, losses of friends and family, and anticipation of one's own death; and (3) creative expression which fosters an increase in self-esteem and autonomous functioning.

The structure of the art groups is open-ended, emphasizing individual choice of materials and subject matter. The purpose of this format is to enable group members to focus on and share their concerns of the moment, to foster independent decision making, and to accommodate varying levels of ability and areas of interest. Pre-planned projects are less frequently employed. When utilized, they are designed to be flexible, encouraging spontaneity and variations of individual preference.

The success of this kind of free-choice format is dependent upon a consistent, supportive structure imposed by the group leader. The elements of this crucial underpinning of the activity are consistency of group meeting day, time, place and membership; an adequate, but not overwhelming choice of appropriate materials, and most importantly, the guidance of the art therapist. A trained art therapist can make interventions which are based upon a knowledge of group dynamics, the creative process, technical use of the art media, and aspects of psychological and cognitive functioning relevant to the population served.

THE ROLE OF THE ART THERAPIST

The first task of the art therapist is to provide an environment in which the creative process can flourish. This means as much privacy for the group as possible, a spacious work surface, adequate lighting and freedom from noise, interruptions and other distractions. The art therapist must be able to motivate participants to try the activity and to keep working. The art therapist helps with decision making and problem solving by offering possible solutions which the participant may choose to accept or reject. If necessary, more active support is offered, for example, starting a drawing, mixing colors of paint, or rebuilding a collapsed clay construction. Such intervention is appropriate when it fosters the creativity and independence of the individual.

The art therapist acknowledges the accomplishments evident in the art work, affirming the unique abilities of each participant. Respect must be shown for the art product and the person who made it by carefully storing and protecting it from being damaged or discarded. Whenever possible, the completed work is attractively displayed where it can be viewed by the art group and others.

The most effective art materials are those which are not difficult to begin to use, are simple enough to enable completion of a work within a short period of time, and can communicate what the participant wishes to convey quickly and directly. Materials should be sturdy, attractive, well-maintained, and not difficult for use by those who may have arthritis, limited grip strength, reduced vision or other physical impairments. Oil pastels, tempera paint and drawing pencils are essential. If a kiln and adequate facilities for storage and clean-up are available, clay is a wonderful medium. Also useful are felt tipped markers, chalk pastels, colored pencils, watercolors and collage materials. Methods of adapting materials for use by those with severe motor impairments have been described by Katz and Katz (1987). For example, brushes may be made easier to grip with the addition of materials such as wooden dowels and strapping tape. Adaptational aids can be created to allow brushes to be attached to the foot or head, or held in the mouth. Paint jars can be prevented from spilling by anchoring them in a weighted kitchen spice rack.

Older persons with mental retardation sometimes exhibit behaviors more suited to younger persons, in conformance with what has been expected of them. Having frequently resided with, and worked with, younger adults, they may not have acquired a realistic concept of their own chronological age. Media associated with children, such as crayons or finger paint, are therefore counterproductive in fostering age awareness. They also detract from the sense of dignity necessary to an optimal level of independence.

Craft materials as they are traditionally employed are not usually well suited for an art therapy program. Craft work emphasizes adherence to specific techniques and to a series of steps which must be followed to assure success. The end product, a useful, functional object, is the ultimate goal. Art work is usually neither useful nor functional. In art as therapy, the process is more important than the product. There is no right or wrong way to proceed. Success depends more upon experimentation, imagination and allowing one's own uniqueness to take center stage. Communication of thoughts or feelings is more readily facilitated by drawing materials, for example, than by weaving. For these reasons, craft materials may be associated with tasks which are inconsistent with the goals of art therapy. If present in the art therapy area, participants may immediately gravitate to them because they are seen as less difficult to use than "fine art" materials.

MOTIVATION

Many of the residents were not accustomed to participating in group activities. Some were unacquainted with art materials. One man told me, "You'd have to be smart to make pictures like that," perhaps fearful of revealing cognitive deficits. Another man made clear that getting a job was much more important to him than painting. A few were eager to try, but frequently abandoned sessions after a brief attempt at drawing. How could this disparate group of individuals be engaged, counteracting the fear and apathy which were so ingrained from lifelong experience?

Challenge and risk-taking are an inherent part of making art, or pursuing any creative activity. Where this is anticipated, a fear of failure may ensue. It is further compounded by the experience of persons with mental retardation, who may have felt inadequate and frustrated on many occasions. Therefore, it is important both to establish a sense of safety and security, and to present the activity in such a way that some successes can be achieved relatively quickly.

Rather than overprotection, an environment of emotional safety is one of consistent non-judgmental acceptance and reassurance. The group leader communicates that participation is always voluntary, that no one will be pushed to do something he or she does not want to do. Respecting the right to self-determination of the older adult is crucial to the task of eliciting independent initiative. This initiative is essential to creative activity.

Safety is also established when the group leader can communicate that the members' art work will never be rejected, regardless of its content, and that the verbal expression of feelings, negative or positive is welcomed. A woman who participated sporadically appeared to be reluctant to join the group on a particular morning. The art therapist reminded her of the "beautiful" picture she had made on a previous occasion. She immediately replied that if she made a picture today, it wouldn't be beautiful, relating her anger at another resident. When the therapist encouraged her to express her mood and make an "unbeautiful" picture, she did so. The resulting work was a breakthrough for her in that she was able to use human imagery for the first time.

Those who are clear in their refusal to do art work can be encouraged to sit with the others and talk and watch. If this can be accomplished, they can usually be gently directed into some kind of tentative exploration of the art materials. However, very resistant persons will keep physically distant from the others. Here it is important for the group leader to establish an ongoing relationship so that trust can slowly develop. With one such individual, the art therapist took an interest in his needlework projects, pencil sharpener collection, etc., talking to him without demanding participation. Eventually the therapist's acceptance of and interest in him motivated him to begin making pictures.

Once an individual has begun working, an important hurdle has been overcome. However, motivational techniques are necessary to keep people engaged when they become discouraged or when they just don't know what to do next. Rather than jumping in to fix things or to offer reassurance, it is important to find out what it is that is causing the difficulty. Questions such as "What part of the work do you like here?" or "What is it that you don't like here?" convey that the picture or sculpture as a whole need not be rejected, and that making decisions about what works and what doesn't is part of the process that all artists undertake.

A few of the participants quickly covered the page with letters, lines, circles, etc. and then, almost compulsively, went on to do the same on numerous subsequent sheets of paper. For these individuals, intervention is eventually necessary in order to foster some artistic development and interrupt the cycle of repetition. They can be slowed down by giving them larger sheets of paper and steering them away from "fast" media such as paint. They can be encouraged to elaborate on simple designs by placing smaller circles within larger ones, for example, or to cover all the white spaces on the page with color. Others may make one image in the center of the page and say they are finished. The participant has a right to determine when a work is complete. However, questions such as, "What might be around the outside of the house?" or "What kind of weather/time of day/season might it be?" will sometimes inspire the expansion of the subject matter and make a richer composition.

RESPONDING TO THE ART WORK

The art therapist or other staff person's comments about the work as it progresses and is completed will inevitably have some impact on the outcome of the experience for the older adult. Responses which will encourage the participant to keep developing his or her personal vision are those that show a genuine interest in the participant's own perceptions of the work as well as in the process which was undertaken to create it. For example, one might ask, "Is there anything you would like to tell me about that house that you've put so much work into?" or say, "I noticed you decided to use colored pencil instead of pastel. Which one seems to work best for you?" Helpful responses acknowledge the uniqueness of the work and de-emphasize the importance of relying on external opinions. Even if it is heartfelt, general compliments (such as "That's lovely") are less effective than noting specific areas of strength. When one man drew some flowers, the art therapist noted that he had used three different ways of making the blooms in his picture. The intent was to encourage his tendency to experiment and to help him realize there is no one "right way" to do things in art.

Because of the nature of art education at the time, any early experience with art which older persons with mental retardation had in school or institutional settings was likely to have emphasized representational or realistic rendering of objects. In order to foster a free enjoyment of the art materials and to accommodate persons whose level of impairment prohibits them from making recognizable imagery, this kind of preconception must be overcome. A passing staff member may approach an individual working on an abstract design and ask, "What is that?" In this instance, the individual is left feeling confused and judged. Instead of trying to make a recognizable image, he or she may have been energetically exploring the properties of color and composition.

FOSTERING AUTONOMOUS BEHAVIOR

Many older persons with mental retardation, whether having spent life in an institution or cared for by family, are accustomed to having their decisions made for them. They may tend to act frequently on the basis of what is expected of them, or what will please those on whom they are dependent. In order to function independently to the degree possible within the limitations of mental and physical impairment, the individual must be able to become aware of and express preferences. Art activities are an excellent context for practicing the important skills of identifying one's needs and desires, taking the responsibility for making choices which one is capable of making for oneself, and using assertive, socially acceptable behavior to pursue one's goals.

These large tasks can begin in very small ways, for example, in exercising the option of where to sit, what size paper to draw on, how long one will work, etc. In the beginning, individuals may need assistance and encouragement in making these basic choices. The group leader can reinforce independent behavior for those who are particularly passive by noting any deliberate action taken ("I see you decided to change to a new color."). He or she can also help by asking questions about wishes, likes and dislikes, even if they cannot at first be answered. Open-ended questions, rather than those requiring a yes or no response, are most effective. When group members perceive that there is an interest in and acknowledgment of their preferences, they will begin to respond accordingly.

ART AND DEVELOPMENTAL ISSUES

Despite the fact that elders with mental retardation face losses and the anticipation of their own deaths just as do nondisabled elders, caregivers have traditionally "protected" them in the belief that their understanding of death is too limited to openly encounter this subject (Kultgen, Rinck & Pfannenstiel, 1986). However, a study described by Lipe-Goodson and Goebel (1983) showed that adults with retardation have a higher awareness of death than would be indicated by IQ alone; they have learned from experience. At whatever level an individual is capable of understanding, he or she is entitled to explore feelings and preconceptions about this important issue. Where loss has already occurred, lack of this kind of opportunity may result in depression, anxiety or aggressive behavior.

Once the group has become attentively absorbed in the nonverbal task of creating art, they will begin to talk to the group leader and to each other about their concerns. Or, they may express them through the content of the artwork. If the leader encourages any communication of ideas, fears and wishes about health, the death of friends or family members, what they expect will happen to themselves, etc., these topics will come to the forefront. For example, one resident said she thought it was her own fault that her mother had died. She said she wished she had been able to continue living at home with her. The woman next to her responded, "When it's time for her to die, she has to die." A man who has limited verbal skills added, "I'm going to die too."

Reminiscence is also a crucial developmental task. Older persons are often so eager to talk about their memories that the group leader's expression of interest and occasional questions are enough to get things started. It is important to be receptive to reminiscences tinged with sadness, anger or other negative emotions as well as more positive emotions. Older persons with mental retardation may not have had sufficient opportunity to share the distressing aspects of growing up with a mental disability in our society. Many of the memories surfacing in the art group described here were unpleasant ones. For example, some of the residents described responses to their behavioral difficulties which entailed being restrained or given

injections "to put me to sleep." Others described some very difficult family situations they experienced before being institutionalized. Happier memories have also emerged, for example, of a parent who was remembered as nurturing, or of the satisfaction of
earning some money of their own.

CRISIS INTERVENTION

When activities are designed with sufficient flexibility to accommodate the "here-and-now" situation, unexpected events can be
processed therapeutically within the art group. On one occasion, the
art therapist arrived to find that one of the residents had been hospitalized due to a downturn in the course of his terminal illness. It was
suggested that the group write (or dictate) letters, and/or make pictures to send to the hospitalized man. Before the formation of the art
therapy group, distress was expressed indirectly and behaviorally.
It was not until they were given a structured opportunity that the
participants were able to articulate some of their feelings about the
absent resident and the frightening context of his departure.

On another occasion there had been physical conflict between
two of the residents earlier in the day of the art session, and the
entire group was agitated. Extra staff persons were massed to inter-
vene if necessary. Sensing that the participants were not capable of
their usual level of creative effort due to the stressful events of the
morning, the art therapist changed her style as a group leader. She
became an active, supportive participant, doing some drawing with
and for the individuals who requested such assistance. In this instance, being a facilitator was insufficient, and challenging the participants to take artistic risks would have been counterproductive.

IMPACT OF THE ART THERAPY EXPERIENCE

The impact of the residents' participation in the art group has
been assessed by informal interviews with the group home staff,
observation of the residents' attendance and functioning within the
group over time, the residents' comments about the art experience
and the art therapist's examination of the art products. Staff report
that, 7 months after the start of the program, the residents have a

greater readiness to explore their own capabilities, that they are more self-confident and more likely to "jump right in" to new activities. Staff also note that there has been an increase in initiative-taking and expression of preferences, especially in the case of some individuals who were particularly passive.

An increase in positive comments by residents about their own art work as well as that of others has been observed, reflecting greater self-esteem. Increased social interaction and group cohesion have been apparent on occasions where residents have shared pictorial imagery with each other and drawn each other's portraits. For several individuals, the level of participation and the length of attention span has grown over the course of exposure to the group, which are reflected in frequency of sessions attended and time spent making a particular work.

As described above, therapeutic art experiences have been useful as a productive outlet for anger between residents, as a stabilizing, calming activity during times of crisis, and as an avenue for expression of feelings about loss related to the hospitalization of a resident.

Most concretely, the impact of the art group has been evident in the case of two of the residents who were severely debilitated and bedridden at times, due to depression and cancer, respectively. Despite the fact that these two individuals had not been getting up regularly even for meals, the arrival of the weekly art sessions was a consistent impetus for them to join the other residents in an activity. During periods of crippling emotional or physical pain, they remained able to draw and paint, sharing moments of sadness, humor, and pride in their accomplishments.

CONCLUSION

The project described above was initiated on a pilot basis with a small group of individuals at one site. Based upon the initial success the experience, replication and further development of the concept of this kind of programing must occur. There is a need to refine the approach and to more formally test its efficacy in improving aspects of the lives of older persons with developmental disabilities. The exploratory work having been undertaken, a more systematic method can be devised to collect data which will measure the impact on adaptive behavior and creative development of participants in future projects. Adaptation of the program strategy for use in other settings such as nursing homes, day programs or senior centers is also needed.

This pilot effort also suggests an agenda for training professionals involved in the provision of art therapy services as well as other persons responsible for the care and activities of the participating elders. In order to achieve the maximum beneficial impact of this modality as applied to the population of older persons with developmental disabilities, training needs to occur in the following areas, some of which have been discussed above: (a) aging and disability, (b) awareness of the psychological tasks of older adulthood, (c) the use of art as therapy, (d) cognitive and creative capacities brought to the art-making process by persons with mental retardation, (e) appropriate materials, (f) motivating participation and independent behavior, and (g) handling of, and verbal response to, the art products.

REFERENCES

Jungels, G. (1982). *To be remembered: Art and the older adult in therapeutic settings*. Buffalo, NY: Potentials Development for Health and Aging Services.

Kramer, E. (1971). *Art as therapy with children*. New York: Schocken Books.

Kultgen, P., Rinck, C., & Pfannenstiel, M. (1986). *Training guide for aging specialists*. Kansas City: UKMC Institute for Human Development.

Kunkle-Miller, C. (1978). Art therapy with mentally retarded adults. *Art Psychotherapy, 5*, 123-133.

Lipe-Goodson, P. & Goebel, B. (1983). Perception of age and death in mentally retarded adults. *Mental Retardation, 21*(2), 68-75.

Ludins-Katz, F. & Katz, E. (1987). *Freedom to create*. Richmond, CA: Institute of Art and Disabilities.

Naumburg, M. (1973). *Introduction to art therapy: Studies of the "free" art expression of behavior problem children and adolescents as a means of diagnosis and therapy* (rev. ed.). New York: Teachers College Press.

O'Malley, W. (1983). Art therapy with the mentally impaired. In A. DiMaria, E. Kramer, & E. Roth (Eds.), *Art therapy: Still growing. Proceedings of the 13th annual conference of the AATA* (pp. 32-34). Alexandria, VA: American Art Therapy Association.

Rubin, J. (1984). *The art of art therapy*. New York: Brunner/Mazel.

Rugh, M. (1985). Art therapy with the institutionalized older adult. *Activities, Adaptations & Aging, 6*(3), 105-120.

Weiss, J. (1984). *Expressive therapy with elders and the disabled: Touching the heart of life*. New York: Haworth Press.

Wilson, L. (1977). Theory and practice of art therapy with the mentally retarded. *American Journal of Art Therapy, 16*, 87-97.

Chapter 6

ART AND CRAFTS –
Not "Arts and Crafts" –
Alternative Vocational Day Activities
for Adults Who Are Older
and Mentally Retarded

Rae Temkin Edelson

SUMMARY. Often "arts and crafts" – a somewhat pejorative recreational term – is seen as part of a service base for older adults with
and without developmental disabilities. An alternative age integrated vocational day activity with salesworthy art and fine hand
crafts as a program base is described. This program model can provide meaningful work for older persons with mental retardation on a
part to full-time basis that can lead into meaningful avocational activities along with changing needs as individuals age. The image-
enhancing effect of art based activities can enhance self-images under siege by the double stigmas of old age and disability.

People with developmental disabilities and mental retardation are
living longer than ever before (Rancourt, 1989). Where should
these individuals live? Where should they go during the day? Community based programs for living, adult education and meaningful
day activities are proliferating for the older segment of the population. Catapano, Levy and Levy (1985) and Janicki (1988) warn

Rae Temkin Edelson, MA, MS, is Program Director of Gateway Crafts, a
Vinfen Corporation Program in Brookline, MA, which is funded by the Massachusetts Department of Mental Retardation.

against premature retirement for older adults with mental retardation. They suggest that regression to custodial care may occur unless other activities replace the individual's previous work or day program experience. Age bias is a challenge and stigma that faces older adults (Erikson, Erikson and Kivnick, 1986). Older adults with mental retardation face the double stigma of age and disability.

In considering what options older people who are mentally retarded should have for their day activities it seems clear that programs based on art and fine hand crafts can have a significant place in vocational day activities. Art based activities of high quality often have a halo effect on social acceptance and self esteem as they build skills. Thus, these activities may be tools in reaching what Wolfensberger (1983) cites as the highest goal of normalization: creating and supporting valued social roles for people who are at risk of social devaluation (p. 234).

THE ROLE OF ART BASED VOCATIONAL ACTIVITIES

Seltzer (1988) states that 76% of older community residence members with mental retardation have no day placement. The majority who do have day placement participate only in basic and unchallenging day activities. Catapano, Levy and Levy (1985) stressed that a broad range of day activities should be provided for these individuals including day activity, recreation, and specialized employment. De Brine and Howell (1989) indicated that work for pay is essential for self esteem. This is particularly so for older individuals with mental retardation who may be at risk of social devaluation.

If work activities are critical in the menu of services for some older adults with mental retardation, then what type of work is most suitable? Seltzer (1988) suggested that modifications should be made in the vocational activities provided for older individuals with mental retardation with particular attention being paid to age appropriateness, and to the provision of suitable levels of support. Activities in settings which are integrated with respect to age are also stressed (Catapano, Levy and Levy, 1985). The goals of such activities should include efforts to develop motor and self-care skills and prevent their regression, (Catapano, Levy and Levy, 1985). It is also important to exhibit flexibility in terms of people's attendance and to emphasize strengths and abilities.

Art-based services can play a crucial role in this continuum of vocational activities for older individuals with mental retardation. Art and crafts are certainly respected activities for older adults in the general population and are a staple of adult education courses and program activities in senior citizen facilities. Erikson and Erikson (1986) suggested that art, perhaps neglected in youth, can enrich old age and enhance sensory involvement. While this is important for the general aging population, it is especially important for individuals who are aging and mentally retarded.

THE IMPORTANCE OF QUALITY ART

Not everyone who is old will participate in art activities. However, it seems clear that a significant percentage could benefit from such activities. It should be noted that producing high quality art is both possible and desirable for older individuals. Lewis (1987) warns against low quality art, which is too often found in centers for the elderly. He encourages fine art activities of quality. Grandma Moses, who started painting in her late seventies, is an outstanding example of an older adult who flourished in this area of endeavor.

However, staff who facilitate art and crafts programs for individuals with mental retardation, both young and old, too often tend to be satisfied with the production of art with little or no intrinsic value. This tendency has given art programs for the disabled a bad name. For example, Catapano, Levy, and Levy (1985) suggested avoiding arts and crafts activities for older adults with mental retardation. Instead they would offer meaningful experiences involving manual skills that are designed to develop fine and gross motor coordination, perception, and creative expression. When art and crafts are not demeaned as activities, they are generally classified as recreational rather than vocational (Seltzer,1988). Given that art-based activities promote these very skills, it is unfortunate that the field often fails to recognize their potential value.

There can be significant vocational as well as recreational benefits for older individuals with mental retardation who participate in structured and supportive art programs which generate high quality products. The remainder of this chapter will describe one such program.

THE GATEWAY APPROACH

Gateway Crafts is a prevocational training program of the Vinfen Corporation, a large non-profit human services corporation based in Boston, Massachusetts. The program is funded by the Massachusetts Department of Mental Retardation. Gateway provides services for twenty eight individuals with a primary diagnosis of mental retardation. This group includes eleven older adults (age 55 and up) who participate in the program on at least a regular part-time basis. The median age of the older clients at Gateway is 61.1 years. Their median score on the Wechsler Adult Intelligence Scale is 53.6. The guiding belief of the program is that older adults with mental retardation can participate in and benefit from art-based vocational activities.

The setting for the Gateway program is a loft space with natural north lighting. The facility includes a small crafts shop where products made at Gateway are sold to the public. Program members are paid on a piece work basis for items sold.

METHOD

The program at Gateway is two-tiered. The vocational component offers training in fine art (such as water color), ceramics, paper graphics (including card and wrapping paper design), weaving, fabric printing, and silk screening. In the vocational component of the program, the professional level of the art or craft product is stressed, saleability is emphasized, and production goals are developed. Most members of this program component attend five days a week for a six-hour day.

The vocational component of the program offers the same elements and differs only in that it does not emphasize productivity. Although saleabilty is stressed, program participation is also more flexible. Individuals may attend from a minimum of six hours a week up to the full five day week program. Placement in either program component is based on ability, not age.

In addition to these vocational elements, other educational and recreational activities are available to program members. These include weekly exercise groups, trips into the community, and training in self-advocacy, nutrition, and health. Specific schedules for program members are elective and are derived from semi-annual individual goal plans developed by a team of practitioners, family members, and the client. Modifications to the program can be made to accommodate changing medical and personal needs by reconvening the team.

STAFFING AND TRAINING

The program goal of Gateway is to fully use the abilities and interests of the program members in order to develop the highest possible level of art work and fine hand crafts. The measure of the quality of the work is its marketability and its adherence to accepted professional standards. Special instruction in crafts, drawing, and painting is provided. Individuals are exposed to professional crafts and to fine art through the work of recognized artists whose styles relate to the experience and artistic approaches of the program members.

Furthermore, Gateway staff members have a professional background in either artisanry or fine art. Such an approach to staff selection is urged by Lewis (1987) who stresses the use of qualified artists and art teachers as instructors in teaching art to older adults. Erikson and Erikson (1981) suggest that older adults be exposed to art as a profession rather than simply as an avocation. The emphasis is on art as work, rather than on art as therapy or hobby, and the proper role for staff is artist rather than therapist or recreation coordinator.

Gateway staff members are recruited from the body of local artists, artisans and art teachers in the Boston area. The program's priority in staff selection places professional art credentials first and experience in geriatrics and special needs second. Training in working with people who are older and mentally retarded is provided onsite and through inservice training by Vinfen Corporation and the Massachusetts Department of Mental Retardation. The role of the staff is critical in terms of educating, role modeling, and setting professional standards. Having a professional staff facilitates the sale of items, the arrangement of exhibits, and the selection of a product line. Staff members also assist in marketing, through their own existing professional networks.

GATEWAY CLIENT PROFILES

Gateway clients are in the "young-old" category of elderly individuals, with intellectual functioning. Some clients came to the program with significant artistic backgrounds and interests, while others were later identified by the trained staff as having significant ability in fine arts or hand crafts. All, however, are able to do vocational crafts as a day activity and to produce saleable items for which they are paid on a percentage basis.

Although one older man has reduced his program time by one day a week, two other elderly individuals have each increased their schedules by one day a week. Attendance is excellent and none of these individuals fall below the 85 percent attendance requirement set by the Department of Mental Retardation.

A.D., Gateway's oldest client, is 72 years old and a former resident of Monson State Hospital and Fernald State School where he lived from the ages of 4 to 57. He functions in the moderate range of retardation, and has orthopedic difficulties which result in limitations in ambulation. A. received some training in weaving while he was at Fernald. When he was deinstitutionalized he initially worked for one year in a traditional assembly type workshop. He then transferred to the newly formed Gateway program in 1974 and has remained there for the past 16 years. He now lives independently in the community. Although he has been offered other work opportunities he has chosen to remain at Gateway where he has developed great expertise as a weaver. He has expanded his skills over the years and has successfully exhibited his work at local juried crafts fairs. He is an accomplished weaver who does yardage on a subcontract basis with local professional weavers. He is aware that he is old enough to consider retirement, but he has chosen to continue to practice his craft at Gateway, working on a three day a week schedule rather than the five days a week he worked when he was younger. (See Picture.)

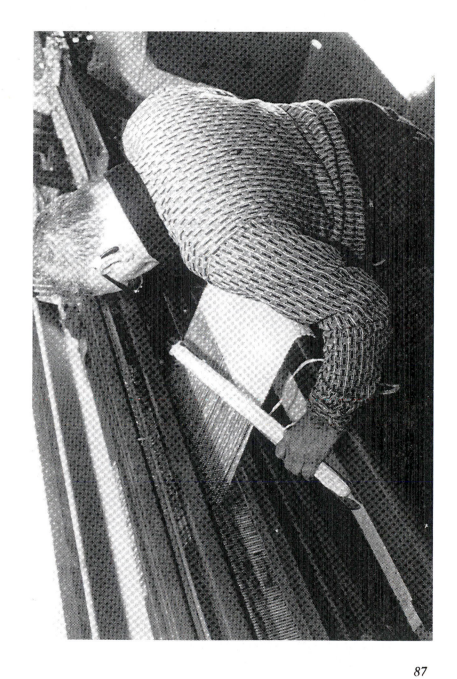

B.H.W., aged 55, lived with relatives in Hong Kong for many years without receiving formal services. He emigrated to the United States in 1966, and lived in a nursing homes from 1967 until 1983. Prior to his acceptance at Gateway in 1979, he had not worked, but did draw as a hobby. He functions in the moderate range of mental retardation. At the beginning of his programming at Gateway he exhibited many somatic complaints, and was not able to work full time. He now lives in a supervised apartment in the community, attends the program full time and is one of Gateway's most publicly recognized individuals. His work has been reviewed in the *Boston Globe* on a number of occasions. He has exhibited at the Cavin Morris Gallery in New York City, a prestigious dealer in "outsider art" — quality art by individuals who are generally lacking in formal art training (Cardinal, 1972). His work is characterized by anthropomorphic drawings, in which a variety of inanimate objects ranging from fruits and vegetables to household appliances are transformed into engaging beings often dressed in the glamorized fashion of old-time Hollywood stars. His original drawings are presented as paintings, cards, and on a product line of mugs, t-shirts and aprons. (See Figure 1.)

ADAPTING MATERIALS AND METHODS

Program members at Gateway have a variety of special needs: deficits in overall intellectual functioning, specific cognitive disorders, visual impairment, and motor dysfunction, ranging from weakness, to low speed in manual tasks and ambulation.

Many of the older adult program members have significant visual losses. The Gateway setting provides ample natural light which assists those with current functional vision. The use of bright colors in program member's art and fine hand crafts enhances the range of activities available to individuals with mild to moderate visual impairment. Ceramics and weaving, due to their tactile nature, are both highly suitable to people who are legally blind. Where little functional vision or poor color sense is present, weaving shuttles of varying length, each with different colors on them are used to create complex patterns. Ceramics can readily be taught to individuals with visual deficits, who often have heightened tactile abilities.

FIGURE 1

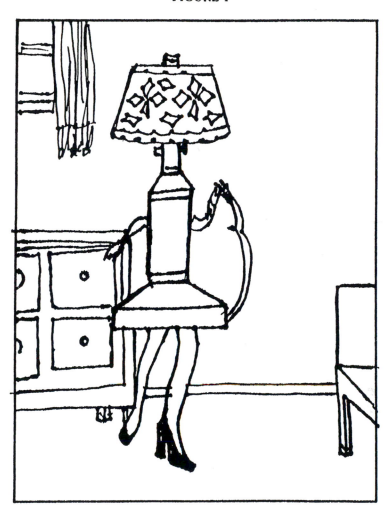

Hand building with clay coils and with clay pressed into molds are skills that can be developed through hands on instruction. Verbal directions, and the use of physical models are particularly helpful in guiding the creation of the final product for individuals who are visually impaired.

For people with poor hand strength or poor motor co-ordination, ceramics can help build vital skills. Manipulation of the clay can build motor abilities. The malleability of clay allows individuals with poor motor skills to correct mistakes in construction without ruining products and experiencing the additional frustration of making irrevocable errors. Items can be clamped in weaving to achieve greater stability. Rubber pencil grips (available through educational supply houses) make holding drawing instruments easier for individuals with poor motor skills and limited hand strength. When paintings on paper or fabric are being executed, the area beyond the scope of the art work can be masked off with a paper template, so that people with poor motor control will not mar a drawing by overshooting the target field. It is well worth the effort to provide these adaptations so that the drawing and manipulative activities inherent to the crafts and art activities can then help build fine motor skills while developing and sustaining any residual visual abilities.

Small classes are provided (one to eight ratio) with individualized instruction available through volunteers and local work study students from neighboring universities. It is particularly important when teaching new tasks to provide the one-to-one instruction necessary for people with significant learning disabilities and cognitive deficits. When task analysis accompanied by review of the individual's historical assessments is insufficient to teach new tasks, additional consultation in the form of an occupational therapist's assessment may be obtained, in conjunction with follow-up individualized teaching. With older adults, it is critical to devote one's energies toward enabling the individual to do a task through adaptations geared to his/her abilities.

Great attention is also paid to psychological aspects involved in adjusting to work and developing new skills. It is critical to differentiate between functional inability to perform a task and what Jefferson (1987) refers to as the learned helplessness of many older individuals. The high level of anxiety many older individuals exhibit in new situations (Jones, 1980) is dealt with by building on those strengths which are identified in initial evaluations, and by introducing only one new activity at a time. Thus, each day provides guaranteed success as well as a stretch into new activities and skills. Repeating activities and allowing sufficient time for project completion are essential elements in the design of the program.

These methods provide opportunities for learning and success which will enhance poor self images and encourage individuals to attempt and master new tasks.

Many older adults with mental retardation come to the program with preconceived ideas about art and art activities. Some see these activities as childish and require the validation of exposure to professional art work and art history to change this attitude. Most older adults (Jones, 1980) favor photographic realism as a style. This preference is frequently not in line with their abilities, which may involve more abstract work. The satisfaction of doing an abstract work on a handpainted card and seeing it sell can begin to eliminate this attitude and help to prepare the person for more concerted efforts in abstract art.

However, when an individual with mental retardation does display a talent for more realistic rendering, working in Grandma Moses' style has great potential for them; it can bring not only personal satisfaction but a measure of recognition from the professional art world (Jones, 1980).

Many older adults have established patterns of doing needlework or latchhook prior to joining a program. This can be expanded on by encouraging them to draw original designs for embroidery or latchhook, rather than using kits. This allows them to make saleable handcrafted items which are unique.

Other essential provisions for older adults involve allowing sufficient time to move around the program space, clean up, store materials and gather one's possessions before leaving. A slow, steady pace is encouraged for older program members who have difficulty with ambulation, and speed.

A variety of adaptations for the older adult with mental retardation must be made based on the characteristics of that individual; personality traits, abilities, interests, specific deficits in vision, motor ability, learning style and cognitive and learning deficits. Because of the broad range of activities outlined in the vocational art program, a wide variety of older individuals with mental retardation and other special needs should be able to succeed if the necessary adaptations are made.

PROGRAM EVALUATION

Table 1 outlines the methods used to measure progress in the vocational crafts program. Evaluation at Gateway is in its incipient stages, and it is too early to have results. However, the table delineates the relevant variables to measure and suggests means for collecting information on these variables.

All evaluative material is gathered in a manner suited to the item being tracked, with data and work samples collected on a daily to weekly basis as products are completed. Exhibits and fairs are logged as they take place. Press clippings and photographs are filed to measure progress and distributed to further community awareness.

Gateway's data collection sheets and progress notes document that program members have shown improvement in both skills and sales. Similar gains in crafts skills have been shown with institutionalized elderly (Weiss, Schaefer, Forrest, 1989), where improvement in fabric techniques was shown to increase along with significant social interactions gains. It is particularly noteworthy that overall crafts sales at Gateway have risen from $800 per year in 1977 when the program had 12 full time members, to a current $20,000 per year with membership of part and full time members at 28.

ART AND SOCIAL STIGMA

Art has an established historical and cultural value, and a wealth of positive associations that can enhance and upgrade the images of individuals who are active participants in the art world. Art therefore can break through stereotypes of mental retardation, old age, and the resulting social stigma. Taylor (1987) praises the effect that art has in counteracting the negative experience of ageism.

Gateway participants engage in juried exhibitions and sell at craft fairs, on site and through other retail locations in the greater Boston area. People who see and buy work by older Gateway artists and artisans have the opportunity to view them as skilled individuals first, and people who are older and with disabilities second. The effect of appreciating these accomplishments helps to reduce the

TABLE 1. Evaluation

Factor	Elements of Tracking
Art/Crafts Performance	Folders with comparative work samples, photographs of work Data sheets on number of saleable products Dollar amount of sales Exhibits (group or individual)
Community Interface	Sales Exhibits Newspaper articles Television coverage
Attitude	Annual evaluation of program Attendance Social interaction at work site
Self Esteem	Positive/negative statements about themselves Statements about themselves as artists or craftspeople Promotion of their own work Changes in physical appearance at work site Physical appearance at public events

practice of labelling all elderly individuals with mental retardation as "disabled." It allows the public to focus on their abilities, their individual art styles, and their skills rather than on their disabilities. Furthermore, television and media coverage enhance the self images of older program members along with the individual's image in the eyes of family, colleagues and other involved professionals. As Taylor (1987) points out, art is an avenue that can provide social acceptance for older adults. This is also true for older adults who are mentally retarded.

COMMUNITY INTERFACE

One of the benefits of a program that is sales oriented is that it provides ample opportunity for community interface. The sales of crafts made by workers can be promoted on site, through local craft fairs and mail order. It is vital for the vocational program to maintain high standards of product selection. This promotes normalization and acceptance of older craftspersons with mental retardation on the basis of good work, not sympathy. Crafts of low quality do a disservice to craftspersons. High quality crafts based on what workers can do well and what the market will accept should be the aim of the program.

Elder craftsman shops are becoming increasingly popular in the United States (Taylor, 1987). Although attempts can be made to gain acceptance for worker's products if such shops exist in one's community, products can also be marketed to whatever local crafts outlets presently exist in the area.

Exhibits are another respected avenue that should be explored to expose the community to the body of art work being produced. Weiss, Schafer, Forrest (1989) encouraged exhibits of art work coming out of programs with institutionalized elderly individuals. Ridgeway and Spaniol (1989) did this with individuals with mental illness. Such efforts date back to Prinzhorn and Dubuffet with collections and exhibits of so called "outsider art," in their case produced by a specialized category of untrained individuals who were mentally ill (Cardinal, 1972). Very Special Arts, a national organization, organizes festivals and exhibits featuring work by individuals with disabilities.

IMPLICATIONS FOR FUTURE PROGRAMMING

Older adults with mental retardation represent a growing population. In developing service models, professionals should first and foremost respect the individuality of the people for whom programs are designed.

Art-based vocational day activity is one such service model that can be offered as part of a successful program menu. It furthers the goals of maintaining manual skills, enhancing self image and self worth, as well as integrating individuals into the community through sales and exhibits. Such a service can easily serve a heterogeneous population, thus promoting the integration of older individuals through their day program.

This type of program should be flexible in terms of the number of days which program members are required to attend, accommodating changes in health, as well as interests. It provides remuneration for the adult as the person ages and can lead to more avocational pursuits as the person's level of activity decreases with age.

The gentle therapeutic setting of an art-based program, along with the therapeutic nature of art-based activities, provides a critically needed supportive environment for older adults with mental retardation who may have accompanying psychiatric difficulties as well as physical disabilities. The value of making a finished product which can be sold and shared with friends and family also has great importance to the program members.

Programs based in the arts break through stereotypes of old age and mental retardation. The Gateway approach described in this chapter can only be effectively executed if full attention is given to the many essential aspects of an art-based program for individuals with special needs. One must design and administer an art program, operate a small business, and finally, provide a human service institution dedicated to the many changing, challenging, individual needs of the people whom it serves.

For older adults, there is life after retirement. For older adults with mental retardation, there can be a fourth act after school, sheltered workshops, and supported employment. This stage should include vocational day activities based on art and crafts performed at a professional level (see Figure 2). This challenging rehabilitation approach introduces art as a viable, essential option.

FIGURE 2

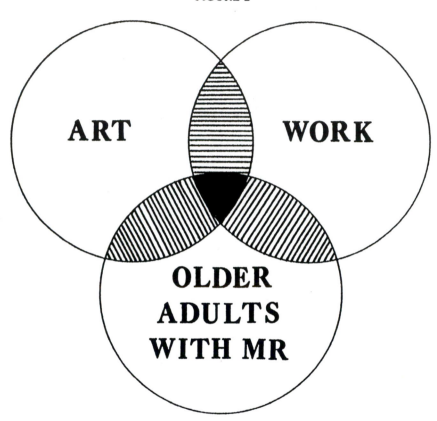

REFERENCES

Cardinal, R. (1972). *Outsider Art*. New York: Praeger.
Catapano, P.M., Levy, J.M., Levy, P.H. (1985). "Day Activity and Vocational Program Services." M.P. Janicki and H.M. Wisniewski (Eds), *Aging and Developmental Disabilities: Issues and Approaches*. Chapter 18, 305-316. Baltimore: Paul H. Brookes.
Debrine, E.J., and Howell, M.C. (1989), "Work and Retirement," in M.C. Howell, D.G. Gavin, G.A. Cabrera, and H.A. Beyer, (Eds), *Serving the*

Underserved: Caring for people who are both old and mentally retarded. 224-232. Boston: Exceptional Parent Press.

Drake, M. (1988). "Art Media with Aging Adults: View from Near the Finish Line." *Gerontology.* 11:3:28-30.

Eilenberg, C. (1989). "Older Artisans for a New Age." *Boston Seniority.* 8-9.

Erikson, E., Erikson, J. (1981). "On Generativity and Identity: from a conversation with Erik and Joan Erikson." *Harvard Educational Review.* 51:2:249-269.

Erikson, E., Erikson, J., Kivnick, H. (1986). *Vital Involvement in Old Age.* New York: W.W. Norton and Company.

Janicki, M.P. (1988). "Symposium Over-view: Aging — The New Challenge." *Mental Retardation.* 26:4:177-180.

Jefferson, M.F. (1987). "Essentials Adult Educational Programs in the Visual Arts." *Art Education.* 40:4:32-41.

Jones, J.E. (1980). "On Teaching Art to the Elderly: Research and Practice." *Educational Gerontology.* 5:17-31.

Lewis, H.P. (1987) "Art and Older Adults: An Overview." *Art Education.* 5-41.

Rancourt, A.M. (1989). "Older Adults with Developmental Disabilities/Mental Retardation: Implications for Professional Services." *Therapeutic Recreation Journal.* First Quarter, 47-55.

Ridgeway, P., Spaniol, S.E.. (1989). *Art and Mental Illness: New Images.* Boston: Center for Psychiatric Rehabilitation, Boston University.

Seltzer, M.M. and Krauss, M.W. (1987). "Community Based Day Programs." *Aging and Mental Retardation.* 79-99. Washington D.C.: American Association on Mental Retardation.

Taylor, C. (1987). "Art and the Needs of the Older Adult." *Art Education.* 40:4:8-15.

Weiss, W., Schafer, D., Forrest, J. (1989). "Art for Institutionalized Elderly." *Art Therapy.* 6:1:10-17.

Wolfensberger, W. (1983). "Social role valorization: A proposed new term for the principle of normalization." *Mental Retardation.* 21:234-239.

Chapter 7

Helping Older Mentally Retarded Persons Expand Their Socialization Skills Through the Use of Expressive Therapies

Robert Segal

SUMMARY. The expressive therapies, which utilize music, art, and creative movement, can be an effective treatment intervention with elderly mentally retarded persons as a means of helping them expand their socialization and communication skills, thereby reducing problems of social isolation and withdrawal.

PSYCHO-SOCIAL ASPECTS OF AGING AND MENTAL RETARDATION

DiGiovanni (1978) reported that the aging process is experienced similarly by both mentally retarded persons and the general population. Both groups are confronted with social problems related to dependency, isolation, low self-esteem and loss of identity. Erickson (1959) proposed that during particular life cycle stages there are social behavioral tasks that confront all individuals, and these tasks must be mastered during the maturational process. He believed that unresolved issues related to specific life cycles, especially those occurring during childhood or adolescence, could interfere with the completion of later life cycles. From this perspective, it is possible

Robert Segal, PhD, is Professor at the Graduate School of Social Work, University of Houston, and practices family and group therapy. He is a consultant in the field of developmental disabilities and presents workshops for clinicians in the use of Expressive Therapies.

that many mentally retarded persons, who may have had difficulties in meeting some social expectations during various developmental cycles due to their limited social and cognitive skills, may need assistance to deal with the complexities of the aging process.

Butler and Lewis (1977) have documented that some of the emotional reactions that the general elderly population experience related to the aging process are feelings of (1) uselessness, (2) isolation, (3) depression, (4) loneliness, (5) helplessness, and (6) anger. One can anticipate that a number of mentally retarded persons may also experience these emotions as they face the aging process due to their unique social situation.

Seltzer and Seltzer (1985) reported that elderly mentally retarded persons need structured community support services due to the aging or death of their parents. Many of these individuals have led fairly isolated lives. This isolation becomes even more pronounced as they become older. Umberson (1988) reported that the lack of social relationships constitutes a major health risk factor for the elderly. She stated that "just having a relationship has the biggest impact on health," (p. 4). While the issues of social isolation and dependency confront the general aging population, these issues appear to be even more problematic for those persons who experience the double jeopardy of being both aged and mentally retarded.

COMMUNICATION AND SOCIALIZATION ISSUES

The issue of communication as it affects the social needs of elderly mentally retarded persons is an important concern. Because of the precarious social position that these individuals hold, they need to be helped to achieve some level of competence with regard to the acquisition and utilization of communication and socialization skills if they are to survive in our complex society. They need to be provided with a social support system that will assist them in their efforts to participate, in a meaningful way, in an environment that often stigmatizes them and which often places barriers to their positive social functioning.

Keane (1972) reported that mentally retarded persons tend to have a higher prevalence of communication disorders than those in the general population. Some of the communication problems that these individuals have may be related to social and emotional factors.

Zigler and Balla (1982) explored the basis for communication problems among this population and found that it is related to: (1) limited opportunity to experience meaningful social communication within their restricted environmental setting, (2) a tendency toward being outer-directed rather than relying on their own resources for direction, and (3) a poor self image and low self-esteem due to a history of repetitive social and cognitive failures. To enhance their social skills, one could provide the mentally retarded with structured and directed opportunities for meaningful and successful social experiences.

"Deinstitutionalization" was promoted in the early 1970's because institutionalization inhibited the social and psychological development of developmentally disabled persons. Segal (1972) reported that while living in the community appeared to be more beneficial for these persons, living in one's parents' home or in a group home also posed socialization problems for the mentally retarded due to the constricting and inhibiting climate in many of these settings. Often parents in their own homes or house parents in group homes demanded conforming behaviors as a way of assuring that the mentally retarded person would more easily "fit" into society, hoping to decrease stigmatization. The result of these well meaning social pressures often reinforced the mentally retarded person's dependency. It is not, therefore, surprising that as some mentally retarded persons experience the aging process, they find it hard to take risks and to be openly communicative, and they become withdrawn. In order to minimize their social isolation, the elderly mentally retarded should have access to programs that would enhance their communication and socialization skills. Recently, socialization programs involving the expressive therapies (art, music, and creative movement, etc.) have been implemented to meet these goals.

GOALS OF EXPRESSIVE THERAPIES

The goals of expressive therapies as a treatment intervention with the elderly mentally retarded are: (1) to encourage them to purposefully interact with others in their environment, (2) to assist them in expressing and communicating their feelings and ideas; and (3) to stimulate their cognitive processes so as to enable them to sharpen their problem solving skills. Additional goals are: (1) to stimulate their sensory and muscular responses, particularly through the use of music and creative body movement, and (2) to encourage the improvement of their gross and fine motor skills, which may occur through their use of musical instruments and the manipulation and use of art materials.

IMPLEMENTING AN EXPRESSIVE THERAPIES GROUP

Prior to the implementation of a group using the expressive therapies, meetings with the administrators, supervisors and staff should be arranged in order to explain the processes that will be used to achieve the group's objectives. It would be helpful if the group leader could provide a demonstration of the techniques that will be used, since some of the staff may be unacquainted with these processes.

It is preferable that group activities be six to eight weeks in duration which would permit the implementation of short term, limited goals. The group should meet at least once a week for one and one-half hours to provide continuity and to sustain group momentum. A shorter time period would not provide sufficient opportunity for in-depth exploration of the members' issues. A longer time frame could strain the attention span and the energy level of most elderly retarded persons. In order to provide individualized attention, the size of the group should be limited. The maximum number should be eight members.

The ages of the group members may vary. Generally, members should be men and women who are at least 50 years of age. While the group could accommodate a mix of classifications, it would operate more effectively if the participants functioned primarily on the same behavioral and cognitive level (mildly, moderately or severely retarded). The primary criteria would be the individual's capacity to function within a group structure. Possessing minimal social and communication skills would also be advantageous.

Group sessions should be held in an enclosed room to assure privacy and quiet. Since some exercises may be carried out on the floor, the room needs to be carpeted as well as large enough to accommodate wheelchairs.

Each session should be carefully planned in order to develop group cohesiveness and continuity. The expressive therapy exercises in the initial sessions should be simple and conducive to producing successful participation. As the group progresses and as the members become more comfortable, the sessions can become more demanding, utilizing more complex exercises. This would involve the group members on a deeper level, both cognitively and emotionally.

SOCIALIZATION AND COMMUNICATION INTERVENTIONS

Through the members' participation in music, art, and creative movement exercises, dysfunctional behaviors, such as social withdrawal and isolation, can be discouraged and extinguished.

Musical Exercises

Being involved in a musical group experience promotes a wide range of positive social behaviors, such as cooperation, attentiveness, patience, and self discipline. Physical withdrawal or social isolation from the group is discouraged. Involvement in the group is reinforced through praise and positive attention.

A musical "follow the leader" exercise can be used to promote social interaction. Group members, sitting in a circle on the floor, are encouraged to select a musical instrument from the center of the circle. Each member, taking turns as a group leader, uses his/her instrument to make a specific musical sound. For example, a member may beat his/her drum consecutively, three times. Each member, in turn, is then instructed to replicate the same three sounds on his/her instrument. This exercise requires the assumption of a leadership role as well as that of a follower and promotes social interaction, social responsibility, and social interdependence. All members are expected to participate in the exercise, and the leader structures the activity in such a way as to discourage withdrawal behavior. The members are verbally rewarded by praise for their participation. They are also asked to share their responses to the exercise. Did they enjoy the exercise? Was it difficult? Was it fun? Which did they prefer, being a leader or a follower? As these reactions to the group experience are shared and as the group discussion becomes more animated, the leader may extend the discussion to other meaningful issues relative to the members' social problems.

Another musical exercise that can encourage the members to verbally share their emotions uses lyrics of purposefully selected songs. For example, the group can be taught a short, simple song that has the following lyrics: "Everybody has feelings. You have to let them show. Everybody has feelings. You've got to let the people know." After the group has learned and sung these lyrics, each member is asked a question related to the concept of the song. Some of the questions posed are: "What makes you happy?" "What makes you sad?" "What frightens you?" "What worries you?" As the group members answer these questions, they are asked to elaborate on the feelings that they expressed. For example, if an individual states that being alone makes him/her sad, he/she is encouraged to tell the group about a specific situation that promoted feelings of loneliness. As the members proceed to describe their current problems, the group leader universalizes these problems (i.e., "Does anyone else in the group ever feel lonely?") and the group, with the leader's assistance, attempts to find solutions to the social problems that are discussed. The group learns that the expression of their feelings is valued and that through the group discussion solutions to their problems may be found. A third musical exercise, teaching the group members the lyrics to a simple song, can be used to encourage the expression of both positive and negative feelings. For example, the members can be taught the popular song, *Sing a Song*, which contains the following lyrics: "Sing, sing a song. Sing out loud. Sing out strong. Sing of good things not bad. Sing of happy, not sad. . . ." Members who may not be able to remember or sing the lyrics are instructed to hum along. This shared activity provides a safe and comfortable opportunity for the group members to express their feelings and ideas and to learn that these feelings are valued. Focusing on the lyrics of the song, the group leader first asks the members to describe in detail the good things that have happened to them during the week. (Some report watching a favorite television show while others describe a trip to a restaurant with family or friends.) After focusing on the positive lyrics of the song, the leader encourages the members to discuss some of the negative events that have occurred. (Because some members have been socially conditioned to repress the expression of negative feelings since such expression may be considered socially unacceptable, they may, initially, resist participating in this part of the discussion.) With the leader's support, the members may describe current negative situations that are troubling them, such as family arguments or fights with friends and the angry feelings that have been aroused. They may also describe social situations in which they felt letdown, which resulted in feelings of sadness or disappointment. When these negative feelings are universalized and accepted, the group cohesiveness can be further strengthened. The members learn that they are not so different from their peers and that they need not feel guilty for having these negative feelings. After the group has reached this level of trust, it is not unusual for them to introduce subjects related to death and their subsequent feelings of grief and bereavement.

Other songs with various themes can be utilized to provoke cognitive and emotional expression. A song, such as *What The World Needs Now*, can stimulate a group discussion related to the human need for love and to feelings of loneliness due to its absence. The song, *Tomorrow*, can be used to explore the idea that the group member need not despair if today seems empty because tomorrow may hold the possibilities for a bright future. Songs can instill hope, and they can serve as a form of catharsis for previously repressed feelings.

Art Exercises

Creating a group mural can be very conducive toward involving the members in a cooperative venture. The group can either sit at a table or on the floor, whichever is most feasible and comfortable, with a large sheet of drawing paper and several boxes of pastel crayons in front of them. They are instructed that as a group they are to draw a picture of what each would like to do on his/her vacation. It may be necessary for the leader to provide considerable assistance and guidance to the members during this exercise. The group members are encouraged to discuss the content and theme of the picture prior to drawing the mural. They are told that each individual's interest regarding his/her choice of vacation should be depicted in the picture even if it is represented by only a symbolic scribble. Members are encouraged to assist one another in the drawing process and to take turns in using the available space on the paper.

In addition to enhancing their socialization skills by this joint venture, the leader can use the art activity to promote group communication by encouraging the members to discuss the content of the completed mural and the meaning of each individual's contribution to the picture.

Another art exercise that promotes the expression of sensitive or "unspoken" feelings is the drawing of family members or friends. For example, the members are asked to draw a sketch of someone they love or like a lot. Often, the pictures that are drawn do not resemble faces or bodies. Sometimes, they are merely scribbles or lines or stick figures. No mention is made of the artistic quality of the picture since the quality of the product is unimportant. Instead, the focus is on whom the picture represents. Each member is asked to provide information about the person that he/she has drawn. Who is the person represented? Why is this person loved or admired? What kinds of activities do the member and this person share? Through a guided discussion, each member is helped to communicate some very important feelings and experiences related to a significant person in his/her life. If there are any problem areas in the relationship, support is provided to help the member share these problems with the group. Efforts are made through the group discussion to determine if solutions to these problems can be found.

A final art exercise that can be used involves the members in molding soft clay representations of themselves. After making the clay figure, each participant is encouraged to talk about the unique characteristics of the figure. Is the figure handsome/pretty? Is the figure strong? What does the figure like to do? Through this discussion, the group members reveal attitudes and feelings regarding their self worth. The exercise serves as a projective technique to evoke verbal discussion. In addition, the act of creating the clay figurine serves as a cathartic experience.

Creative Movement Exercises

Creative movement exercises can be used to promote leadership roles and to foster social interdependence. For example, a movement exercise, "Follow the Leader," can be used to foster leadership and social risk taking. Each member is encouraged to take a turn leading the group in a simple body movement exercise. (This exercise is similar to the childhood game, "Simple Simon Says.") The members are instructed to imitate the chosen leader's movement. Assuming the roles of both leader and follower requires some social skills. After each member has had an opportunity to play the leadership role, the participants are encouraged to discuss their reactions to the activity. They are asked whether they were comfortable or uncomfortable assuming the leadership role. Was it difficult for them to think up a movement for the group to follow? Did they prefer leading the group or following?

Another movement exercise to promote social interaction is "The Interdependent Circle." The group is directed to sit in a circle on the carpeted floor, holding each others' hands as they stretch out their legs in front of them. Individually and consecutively, each member is instructed to move back slowly until the shoulders, back, and head come resting on the floor. This movement is undertaken while each member receives support from the hands of the persons seated to the right and to the left. After the individual has come to a full rest on the floor, he/she is directed to come up slowly to a sitting position with the aid and support from the persons on each side. After every member has had the opportunity to do this part of the exercise, the leader can form diads, triads, and quartets within the group to repeat the exercise while the rest of the group provides the required support. This unique exercise provides the members with opportunities to experience interdependence, intimacy, and trust, all of which are essential to the development of socialization skills. After completing the exercise, the participants are encouraged to communicate their reactions to the activity, thus further reinforcing the positive socialization and communication skills they have acquired. Other kinds of movement exercises, such as simple square or folk dancing, can be used to foster social interdependence.

In addition, exploring different types of creative movements can enable elderly mentally retarded individuals to get in touch with and to express a wide range of emotions, such as joy, anger, fear, and loneliness; some feelings which these adults may have, unfortunately, are repressed or denied which may lead to depression.

As a way to enable group members to get in touch with these feelings, a leader can encourage the group to use simple body movements, such as gliding, skipping, or hopping across the room in time to rhythmic music. An example of the latter is Scott Joplin's bouyant ragtime music. These movements can evoke feelings of freedom. Moving to an Austrian waltz or a Polish polka or an Irish jig can provoke playful, joyous feelings. After the group has moved with some sense of abandonment to this type of music, the leader should encourage the group to discuss the feelings that the movement has evoked and to consider how these feelings are related to their daily life experiences. For example, they can be asked to describe what is happening in their lives at this time that makes them feel happy. Thus, by focusing on the positive aspects of their lives, the members are helped to maintain a more balanced view, thereby minimizing feelings of despair and futility.

A contrasting exercise can be used to help the elderly mentally retarded adults get in touch with repressed feelings of anger, which would be of value since such unexpressed feelings may lead to a state of depression. The group can be encouraged to move spontaneously to music with dissonant tones, such as those composed by Shostakovitch, Prokofiev, or Philip Glass. Heavy metal or rock music with loud, discordant tones may also provoke negative emotions. The leader can initiate and demonstrate various types of body movements that may evoke these types of feelings. Quick, sharp movements of the arms, legs, shoulders, pelvis, back, and head tend to create muscular and emotional tension. Some members may use thrusting arm movements as though they were punching a person or an object. As the participants kinesthetically respond to the music, they are directed to get in touch with their feelings and to relate them to recent life experiences. A follow-up discussion of these experiences helps the members release their pent up emotions. They also learn to accept their negative feelings and to consider possible ways of handling their feelings appropriately.

CONCLUSION

Elderly mentally retarded persons, like their peers, struggle with problems of social isolation and social withdrawal. These dysfunctional behaviors, if left unattended, can lead to depression and despair. Because many elderly retarded individuals have limited communication skills, they find it difficult to express their feelings related to these social problems, further exacerbating their depression. Traditional verbal therapy has not always proven successful with this population. Expressive therapies, involving the use of music, art, and creative movement, focus on symbolic communication, which enables elderly mentally retarded persons to initially express themselves on a projective level. This expression then ultimately leads to a more comfortable and purposeful use of verbal communication. Since there appears to be a direct relationship between socialization and communication, by enhancing the communication skills of elderly mentally retarded individuals through the use of the expressive therapies, their socialization skills can be reinforced and expanded.

REFERENCES

Butler, R. and Lewis, M. (1977). *Aging and mental health*. St. Louis: C. V. Mosby Company.

Di Giovanni, L. (1978). "The elderly retarded: a little known group." *Gerontologist*, 18, 262-266.

Erickson, E. (1959). "Identity and the life cycle." *Psychological Issues*, Monogram I. New York: International Universities Press Inc.

Keane, V. (1972). "The incidence of speech and language problems in the mentally retarded." *Mental Retardation*, 10, 3-5.

Segal, R. (1972, April). "The community placement program: the institution, the resident, and the family." An unpublished paper, presented at the Third Annual Conference. Ann Arbor, Michigan: The Institute for the Study of Mental Retardation.

Seltzer, M. and Seltzer, G. (1985). "The elderly mentally retarded: a group in need of service." *Journal of Gerontological Social Work*, 8, 99-119.

Umberson, D. (1988, July 29). "Health and medicine." *Houston Post*.

Zigler, E. and Balla, D. (1982). "Motivation and personality factors in the performance of the retarded." In Zigler, E. and Balla, D. (Eds.). *Mental retardation: the developmental difference controversy*. Hillsdale, NJ: Lawrence Erlbum Associates.

Chapter 8

Integrating Older Persons with Developmental Disabilities into Community Recreation: Theory to Practice

Barbara Wilhite
M. Jean Keller
Lori Nicholson

SUMMARY. An increasing number of older adults with developmental disabilities are living in community residential settings and in need of community recreation and leisure services. As these individuals move into what is "retirement age" for their demographic cohort, a greater emphasis will be placed on the availability of generic community recreation and leisure services. Characteristics of this growing population of elders, and a rationale for the development of integrated recreation programs are presented. An interdisciplinary model of recreation integration is discussed with implications for therapeutic recreation specialists. The application of this model is illustrated through a case study of an older adult who is developmentally disabled.

Barbara Wilhite, EdD, CTRS, is Recreation Consultant with the Georgia Council on Developmental Disabilities in Atlanta, GA, and serves as Faculty Member for Southern Illinois University at Carbondale in Niigata-ken, Japan. M. Jean Keller, EdD, CTRS, is Associate Professor in Therapeutic Recreation and with the Department of Kinesiology, Health Promotion, and Recreation, University of North Texas. Lori Nicholson, MA, CTRS, is Certified Therapeutic Recreation Specialist with the Department of Therapeutic Recreation at the Shepherd Spinal Center in Atlanta, GA.

Until recently, many persons with developmental disabilities had a relatively short lifespan, lived primarily in public institutions or with their parents at home, and had little interaction with community developmental disabilities service systems (Sison & Cotton, 1989). As a result, their aging was of minor importance (Blake, 1981). As the entire American population has aged, so too has the population of persons with disabilities. In addition, expanding residential options have enabled many elderly persons with developmental disabilities to live in community settings (Roberto & Nelson, 1989).

As these individuals move into what is "retirement age" for their demographic cohort, they may find themselves at a loss. Schedules and plans once determined by their jobs and families should become more self-directed. This period of transition will require a variety of support services, including recreation services. Thus, this relatively new and growing population is receiving increased attention from therapeutic recreation specialists.

This chapter defines developmental disabilities and describes characteristics of the aging population with developmental disabilities. A strategy for integrating this population into recreation services with nondisabled peer groups is presented. Eight steps are included in this comprehensive, interagency integration approach. Application of the integration model is illustrated through a case study.

DEFINITION OF DEVELOPMENTAL DISABILITY

The concept of developmental disabilities first came into use with the passage of the Developmental Disabilities Services and Facilities Construction Act of 1970 (Public Law 91-517). "Developmentally disabled" included disabilities attributable to mental retardation, cerebral palsy, epilepsy, or other neurological conditions, originating before age 18, constituting a substantial disability, and expected to continue indefinitely. In 1975, amendments to the Developmental Disabilities Act (Public Law 94-103) broadened the law to include autism as a categorical disability. Amendments to the Developmental Disabilities Act passed in 1984 (Public Law 98-527) established a functional approach to disability which associated persons with disabilities by common service needs rather than by disability. In addition, the age limit for the origin of the disability was extended to 22 years.

The 1987 amendments to the Developmental Disabilities Assistance and Bill of Rights Act (Public Law 100-146) described further the concept of limitations in function. According to this definition, a developmental disability results in substantial functional limitations in three or more of the following areas of major life activity: (1) self care; (2) receptive and expressive language; (3) learning; (4) mobility; (5) self-direction; (6) capacity for independent living; and (7) economic self-sufficiency (Public Law 100-146, Section 102,5). This definition reemphasized the chronic or lifelong nature of the disability and the need for on-going assistance. The definition of developmental disabilities highlights the major characteristics of persons who would be classified as developmentally disabled.

CHARACTERISTICS OF THE POPULATION

Rose and Janicki (1986) reported estimates ranging from 200,000 to 500,000 persons with developmental disabilities age 60 and over or about 4 out of every 1000 older persons. Ansello and Rose (1989) reported that recent figures suggest this number may be as high as 10 or more of every 1000 persons over age 60. According to Rose (1986), the number of older persons with developmental disabilities is expected to increase significantly in the next 30 years.

Not only is the number of older persons with developmental disabilities increasing, but their life expectancies are increasing as well. For example, 40% of individuals with mental retardation will live to age 60 (Jacobson, Sutton, & Janicki, 1985). Early onset of aging is prevalent, however, among persons with some conditions, primarily Down's Syndrome (Walz, Harper, & Wilson, 1986). Persons with mental retardation with the greatest life expectancies include women, persons who are ambulatory, persons who do not have Down's Syndrome, persons who are less severely retarded, and persons who live in the community (Jacobson et al., 1985).

The health status of older persons with developmental disabilities is generally reported to be similar to that of their nondisabled peers (Stroud & Sutton, 1988). Ansello and Rose (1989) reported that many older persons with developmental disabilities were relatively high functioning, able to communicate, and free of maladaptive behaviors. They however, also stated, that "most older Americans with developmental disabilities have had little education, have been isolated to a great extent from normal life experiences, and have had few relationships outside their immediate family or disabled peer experiences" (p. 9).

As many as 60% of the extremely disabled older population lives outside of institutional settings (Shanas & Sussman, 1981). Two-generation elderly families are increasing with very old parents providing support to an aging son or daughter, or siblings and children of siblings providing care for older relatives with developmental disabilities (Janicki, Seltzer, & Krauss, 1987). As families age, however, the informal support systems of older adults with developmental disabilities diminishes (Seltzer & Seltzer, 1985).

As the graying of Americans with developmental disabilities continues, service providers, along with people with disabilities and their families, must increasingly pursue a quality of life that includes recreation services, activities, living arrangements, social networks, choices, and life opportunities consistent with the abilities of these older persons to interact interdependently within the mainstream of America's communities.

INTEGRATING RECREATION AND LEISURE SERVICE DELIVERY

Rationale

Much of the research conducted on older persons with developmental disabilities has focused on formal services available to and needed by them (Hawkins & Eklund, 1989; Roberto & Nelson, 1989; Seltzer & Seltzer, 1985). Findings have indicated that services needed by older adults with developmental disabilities are similar to those received by older adults without disabilities (Halpern, Close, & Nelson, 1986). Yet confusion, mixed feelings, and general unpreparedness exist as to how to effectively deliver these services (Roberto & Nelson, 1989). As a result, integrated recreation opportunities are not readily available to older adults with developmental disabilities and very little of the literature has discussed this topic (Rancourt, 1989).

"Integration," as defined in the 1987 amendments to the Developmental Disabilities Assistance and Bill of Rights Act, implies the "use by persons with developmental disabilities of the same community resources that are used by and available to other citizens, and participation by persons with developmental disabilities in the same community activities in which nondisabled citizens participate, together with regular contact with nondisabled citizens" (Section 102,5). Accordingly, persons with lifelong disabilities must be assured the same gamut of services available to other older adults. The expectation is that mainstream services, including recreation, will be accessible to *all* elderly persons. While it may be inappropriate to assume that generic recreation services will be appropriate or desirable for all older persons with developmental disabilities, the presence of a disability should not necessarily be viewed as a reason for excluding older persons from the network of community recreation opportunities.

In addition to the legal basis for integrated service delivery, integration of older persons with developmental disabilities into community recreation settings is justified from theoretical and practical perspectives. The application of the principle of normalization (Wolfensberger, 1972; Bank-Mikkelsen, 1969) suggests that recreation and leisure services provide important avenues toward the successful community integration of persons with developmental disabilities (Putnam, Werder, & Schleien, 1985; Beck-Ford, 1981). From an environmental viewpoint, normalization refers to the process of developing culturally appropriate activities and services. From an individual viewpoint, normalization refers to the acquisition of skills necessary for assuming culturally normative social roles and responsibilities (Bajaanes, Butler, & Kelly, 1981). To facilitate the integration process, both the community and the individual in transition must be prepared.

A continuum of recreation opportunities can be created that will enable older persons to experience as satisfying and as independent recreation lifestyles as possible (see Figure 1). This continuum of services includes specialized or segregated programs for individuals with minimum abilities. These individuals require intensive ser-

FIGURE 1. A Continuum of Recreation Opportunities Leading to Integration of Older Persons With Developmental Disabilities

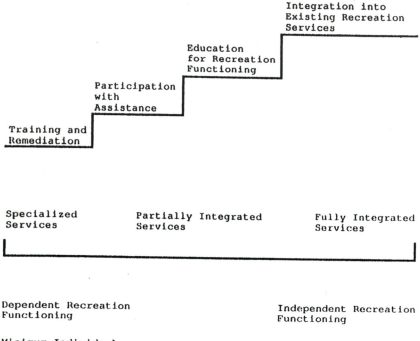

vices that focus on learning and remediation. Partially integrated recreation programs can also be utilized. These programs are less specialized, with an increased focus on developing attitudes and skills necessary for participation in community recreation opportunities. Often these services are physically integrated, that is, they take place in community environments such as bowling alleys, shopping malls, theaters, restaurants, parks, etc. As recreation programs are created to help older persons with developmental disabilities become more interdependent, they can better determine their own level of recreation involvement and integration.

Benefits

Sylvester (1989) suggested that "Community is not just the final destination along the mainstreaming continuum; it is an essential element of quality of life" (p. 20). The challenge for therapeutic recreation specialists is to facilitate recreation services which enable older adults with lifelong disabilities to experience a true sense of belonging or community of spirit; not to just live in a community, but to be socially integrated into that community.

Integrated recreation services provide many benefits to both older persons with disabilities and their nondisabled peers. Access to age-appropriate recreation experiences by older persons with developmental disabilities and nondisabled older persons promotes social interaction, emotional growth, physical development, mental well-being, and helps to break down attitudinal barriers (Krauss & Erickson, 1988).

Integrated recreation activities and services can also provide relief or respite to families and caregivers while at the same time they open up a world of new experiences for older persons with disabilities. Provencal (1988) tells the story of a young social worker having dinner in a nice restaurant with two gentlemen. He asked the men if they had enjoyed their meal. They heartily agreed it was delicious and both said they liked eating in a restaurant. It was their first time. Charles was 60 and Robert was 55. Provencal called for a professional sense of urgency and enjoined service providers to be impatient and adventurous on behalf of their clients.

An Integration Model

Keller (1988) described a strategy for integrating older adults with disabilities into generic recreation and leisure programs (see Figure 2). This strategy begins with the determination of who will participate—consumers and staff members. The characteristics, needs, and abilities of older adults will vary as will those of the

FIGURE 2. Creating a Recreation Integration Process with Older Persons

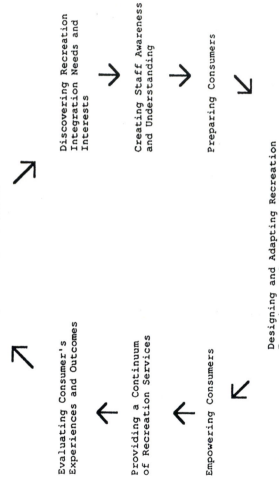

Defining the Target Population
(Consumers and Staff)

Discovering Recreation
Integration Needs and
Interests

Creating Staff Awareness
and Understanding

Preparing Consumers

Designing and Adapting Recreation
Experiences for Successful Integration

Empowering Consumers

Providing a Continuum
of Recreation Services

Evaluating Consumer's
Experiences and Outcomes

recreation, aging, and disability specialists working with them. Time should therefore be taken to carefully identify and select those participants and staff members who will participate in an integrated recreation program.

After the target population has been identified, their recreation needs and interests should be determined. *Step two* of the process explores recreation attitudes, needs, abilities, and interests, and determines the benefits desired from an integrated recreation experience. In-depth interviews and discussions with older adults and leaders of older people with and without disabilities can be utilized to gain this information.

Steps three and four of the recreation integration process involve preparing key players for their roles and responsibilities in assuring community recreation opportunities. These players include personnel from aging, developmental disabilities, and recreation, as well as older consumers with and without disabilities, caregivers, and advocacy groups.

Recreation professionals and community members, disabled and nondisabled older consumers, and families and friends will need to learn about each other and about integration. Recreation professionals will need training on how to provide a wide range of recreation activities and services and ways to adapt or modify present activities and services so that both older adults with and without disabilities will benefit from these experiences (Rancourt, 1989). Older adults with disabilities will need preparation in which personal needs and capabilities are assessed and appropriate levels of activity are determined. Older adults already engaging in recreation programs will also need to be prepared for integration. Some older adults will be reluctant to accept and welcome people with disabilities into their activities (Johnson & Olson, 1982; Kauppi & Jones, 1985). Education about and exposure to older adults with developmental disabilities is essential in preparing the general older adult population for acceptance of integration (Thurman, 1985).

After recreation professionals and consumers have prepared themselves for integration, *step five* of the process emphasizes designing and adapting recreation experiences for successful integration. Consumers must be involved in this process. The likelihood of full integration is reduced when activities are developed *for* rather than *with* participants (Keller, 1988; Taylor, 1988). Input must be obtained regarding the types of activities to offer (e.g., crafts, music, sports, education, volunteer services, travel, etc.) and the preferred methods of delivery. Barriers that affect recreation participation, such as time, cost, location, and transportation problems, should be ascertained. Once barriers are determined, alternatives and modifications can be developed.

Step six in the integration process regards the need to empower older adults with and without developmental disabilities. Recreation professionals will want to tap the abilities of participants, nurture their confidence, help them obtain acceptance, and provide them a strong sense of ownership in activities and services (Keller, 1988). On-going assistance and monitoring from staff may be needed to assure participants are gaining and utilizing skills necessary for interdependent functioning in recreation programs.

Step seven emphasizes the need for an array of appropriate recreation options and the ability to exercise choice. A continuum of recreation services (see Figure 1) provides a variety of activity options ranging in degree of restrictiveness and integration, with a preference for the least restrictive and most normalized setting possible (Taylor, 1988).

The last step in this process regards evaluation of consumers, experiences, and outcomes. However, evaluation should occur throughout the recreation integration process and revisions made at each phase or step as needed. Evaluation questions should relate to the major purpose or goal of each step in the process as well as to the overall success in promoting and sustaining integration. Consumers, recreation professionals, and administrators should be involved in evaluation.

APPLYING THE MODEL

To further describe the process of recreation integration, an application of Keller's (1988) model is illustrated in the case of *Lula Nelson*. Lula Nelson is currently 62 years old and has borderline mild/moderate mental retardation. She lives in a small rural community in central Georgia in close proximity to one of the state's largest cities. Ms. Nelson lived in this community with her mother until she died when Lula was 54. After her mother's death, Ms. Nelson moved in with her younger sister, then 44 years of age, who was divorced with no children. Ms. Nelson's sister worked full-time outside the home.

Ms. Nelson worked at the regional mental retardation service center until age 59. She stopped attending work primarily due to increasing complaints of arthritis, general fatigue, and decreased vision in her left eye due to a blood clot. She resided in her sister's home for the next three years with limited social and recreation involvement. This involvement included visiting, going to church, eating out, and occasionally attending the special social club sponsored by a municipal recreation department in a neighboring large city.

At age 62, with Ms. Nelson's health condition worsening, she suffered a fall in her home. Though Ms. Nelson experienced soreness from the fall, no medical attention was sought. Her sister did, however, arrange for her to receive personal home health care services and assistance with meals three times per week. Unfortunately, six months after the fall, she experienced increasing numbness and weakness in her lower extremities and was diagnosed as having complete paralysis of her lower extremities on her right side and incomplete paralysis on her left side. Ms. Nelson was referred to a private rehabilitation facility by her home health care case manager. Ms. Nelson was admitted to Peachtree Rehabilitation Center in March of 1989.

Determining Direction

After intake interviews and initial assessments, an individualized treatment plan was developed for Ms. Nelson. This plan specified services Ms. Nelson would receive and designated specific staff, family, and community personnel who would be involved in her plan of care. An eight week treatment program was recommended by an interdisciplinary team. These actions illustrate *step one* of the integration process, defining the target population.

Step two of the integration process, discovering needs and defining interests, began by identifying Ms. Nelson's short- and long-term needs relative to returning to her home. Ms. Nelson's treatment plan included occupational therapy for working on activities of daily living such as dressing and personal grooming, and instrumental activities of daily living such as cooking and doing laundry. Her plan also included physical therapy directed toward developing wheelchair mobility and maximizing upper body strength and endurance. Therapeutic recreation was included which emphasized leisure skills building, community reintegration education, and education relative to personal care. Additional efforts in *step two* of the integration process included the development of a separate therapeutic recreation plan by a therapeutic recreation specialist. This plan included leisure/recreation assessment information and goals, activities and leadership methods that would be used to achieve the goals, and a process by which outcomes would be reviewed.

The therapeutic recreation outreach coordinator was assigned to work with Ms. Nelson four weeks prior to discharge. The coordinator and social worker worked together relative to Ms. Nelson's reintegration into her community. Quarterly leisure/recreation outreach clinics and a yearly individualized follow-up meetings were planned for Ms. Nelson following discharge. Ms. Nelson's family and selected community personnel would be included in these clinics. The outreach clinics were viewed as one important avenue for the accomplishment of *steps three and four* of the integration process as they would promote consumer and staff awareness and understanding.

Participation and Education

Ms. Nelson's recreation assessment indicated she spent most of her time at home watching television. She stated that she also enjoyed going out to eat, participating in church services, and attending Young Adult Club meetings. She indicated she had not been very active recently due to her health.

At first, Ms. Nelson appeared frightened of her new surroundings and often withdrew socially to avoid over stimulation. Her initial participation in activities required much encouragement and prompting, sometimes including a personal escort. When given the choice to participate, she often resisted activities.

Assessment information gathered from Ms. Nelson's chart, personal interviews, and observation allowed the therapeutic recreation specialist to surmise that Ms. Nelson's social interaction deficiencies were more a reaction to her recently acquired physical disability and the unfamiliar environment, than a result of inadequate social interaction skills. Thus the specialist began to work with Ms. Nelson to help her understand her current personal attitudes and their affect on her social skills. The therapeutic recreation specialist also worked with Ms. Nelson to reinforce basic social competencies such as introducing herself, maintaining conversations, seeking information, making requests, working cooperatively, and maintaining personal hygiene and appearance.

Ms. Nelson and the therapeutic recreation specialist agreed that assistance provided by a fellow patient would help facilitate her initial activity involvement. In addition, the specialist recognized that utilizing a peer helper could also serve as an appropriate community reintegration strategy that could be recommended at discharge.

Since Ms. Nelson had displayed interest in painting and drawing, the therapeutic recreation specialist decided to introduce her to another patient, Ms. Robinson, who regularly participated in an art group. The specialist asked Ms. Robinson to describe the art group to Ms. Nelson and offer to accompany Ms. Nelson to class, if desired. Ms. Nelson began attending art group with the assistance of Ms. Robinson. She appeared to enjoy the art activities and quickly began to interact spontaneously within the small group. She displayed appropriate social skills and was accepted by her fellow participants.

Ms. Nelson's interest in other activities then began to develop. For example, she had never tried swimming before, and this became a favorite activity. She also enjoyed outdoor activities, particularly fishing. She became a frequent participant in special events.

The therapeutic recreation outreach coordinator first discussed discharge plans with Ms. Nelson and her sister. Ms. Nelson's physical mobility and strength had improved significantly. She still fatigued easily, however, so it was determined that initial involvement outside her home would be limited and increased as her stamina allowed. This approach would also reduce her chance of being overwhelmed by the participation. Thus, emphasis on *step five* of the integration process, designing and adapting recreation experiences for successful integration, began.

Participation in Ms. Nelson's local community senior citizens center was recommended. Ms. Nelson's sister indicated she believed Ms. Nelson preferred attending the Young Adult Club in a neighboring city, but realized how it would be more appropriate and practical for Ms. Nelson to participate in her community with her peer group. Ms. Nelson stated she enjoyed being with the members of the Young Adult Club, but sometimes could not keep up with their pace and simply observed the activities. She expressed both excitement and hesitation over making new friends at a local senior citizens center.

The therapeutic recreation outreach coordinator asked Ms. Nelson if she could contact the community senior citizens center on her behalf. The coordinator explained that she would convey Ms. Nelson's desire to participate in the center's programs and request program information such as brochures and schedules.

The activity director at the senior citizens center responded positively to the therapeutic recreation outreach coordinator's request for program information. The coordinator was then able to discuss with Ms. Nelson general information regarding such things as program activities and center hours and holidays, as well as more specific information regarding registration procedures, fees, wheelchair accessibility, and transportation resources.

The therapeutic recreation outreach coordinator told Ms. Nelson that after she returned home she would begin receiving a quarterly newsletter from the rehabilitation center. This newsletter would inform her of recreation activities and events that were open to former patients. She encouraged her to plan to participate in some of these activities. The outreach coordinator also indicated the date and time of the first quarterly outreach clinic. She explained that these clinics provided an opportunity for her to meet with a therapeutic recreation specialist, other rehabilitation center staff, personnel from the community, and former patients. During this time, Ms. Nelson could discuss successes and problems, receive personal and professional support and encouragement, and obtain technical assistance and resource information.

Community Integration

The recreation integration process was continued upon Ms. Nelson's discharge. After she returned to her home, Ms. Nelson's sister contacted the activity director at the senior citizens center on her behalf. She arranged a meeting between the activity director, Ms. Nelson, and herself. During this time, Ms. Nelson also met the center director and the social worker, and was introduced to a few of the center participants. The activity director discussed daily and weekly center activities as well as special events. She tried to get to know Ms. Nelson and ascertain some of her recreation interests and preferences.

Since Ms. Nelson had developed skills in painting and drawing, she stated she would like to participate in the weekly small group arts and crafts activity. The activity director encouraged Ms. Nelson to attend the arts and crafts class and indicated someone could provide her assistance, if desired. Ms. Nelson also stated she would like to participate in the noon meal and stay for the afternoon socializing session when she "felt up to it." Transportation was arranged for Ms. Nelson to attend the center on Mondays, Wednesdays, and Fridays.

Ms. Nelson indicated she would like to participate in some of the special events, especially if they included fishing. She also expressed her interest in swimming. While this activity was not available at the senior citizens center, the activity director gave her the name and number of the aquatics director at the YMCA in a neighboring large city and encouraged both Ms. Nelson and her sister to contact him. The activity director stated that several of the senior citizens center participants swam at this YMCA and offered to introduce her to these participants.

After this initial meeting, the activity director met with the center director and social worker and discussed ways they could prepare themselves and the other participants for Ms. Nelson's involvement. An educational program involving senior center staff members and participants was planned to discuss mental retardation and spinal cord injury. A part of the educational program included brainstorming potential problems Ms. Nelson and others might encounter. Some of these potential problems were illustrated through role playing. The educational program participants then suggested solutions for these problems. The program participants were encouraged to express their concerns openly. Professionals were available to answer questions and help alleviate concerns.

Center staff decided another action they should take would be to ask Ms. Nelson if she desired a Senior Companion to accompany and assist her during initial recreation participation. Since Ms. Nelson would not be attending the center everyday, the Companion might also be able to visit her at home and provide socialization activities. In addition, they recognized that all of Ms. Nelson's recreation and leisure needs would not be met through her participation in center activities. They realized on-going guidance and encouragement from a variety of service providers and peers would be necessary to empower Ms. Nelson and other center participants, or to accomplish *step six* of the integration process. They vowed to help Ms. Nelson and her sister find and select the most appropriate options.

One of these options was the resumption of home health care services on the days Ms. Nelson did not attend the center. Her home health care aide provided encouragement and assistance as needed relative to personal care and activities of daily living. She also provided companionship, social and intellectual stimulation, and opportunities to expand and refine recreational interests such as painting and drawing.

Providing this continuum of services, as indicated in *step seven* of the process not only helped Ms. Nelson to choose her desired participation options, but also provided her sister with the respite needed to permit her full-time return to work. Through the provision of services including partial recreation integration, recreation participation with assistance, and education for more interdependent functioning, both Ms. Nelson and her sister were able to regain their preferred lifestyles.

The integration process designed for Ms. Nelson will need ongoing evaluation as outlined in *step eight*. Outreach staff from the Rehabilitation Center and aging and recreation staff from the community will need to continue to review and critique their efforts and the effects they have had on Ms. Nelson. They must determine if Ms. Nelson has achieved the intended benefits of services and assess the overall appropriateness of these activities. Revision of individual objectives and/or recreation service design should be made as indicated by evaluation information.

CONCLUSION

Demographic trends suggest there will be a dramatic increase in the number of older adults with developmental disabilities seeking community programs. While their needs will vary, emphasis will be placed on recreation as these individuals move into retirement age. Participation in community recreation programs is their inalienable human and legal right. The task at hand is to insure that there are integrated recreation opportunities available to enhance the quality of their lives.

The acceptance and implementation of integrated recreation programs will not be problem free. Successful programs will probably start small and grow with time and familiarity. As one leader of an integrated Senior Companion program explained, "We are not trying to get our seniors to like and accept all persons with developmental disabilities. We just want them to value, accept, and enjoy the individuals with whom they are involved." A challenge for therapeutic recreation specialists is to design and deliver recreation and leisure services that will enable a growing number of older adults with developmental disabilities to experience a variety of recreation options and achieve a true sense of community using an integration process.

REFERENCES

Ansello, E. F. & Rose, T. (1989). Aging and lifelong disabilities: Problems and prospects. In E. F. Ansello & T. Rose (Eds.), *Aging and lifelong disabilities: Partnership for the twenty-first century* (pp. 9-11). Palm Springs: Elder Press.

Bank-Mikkelsen, N. E. (1969). A metropolitan area in Denmark: Copenhagen. In L. S. Kugel and W. Wolfensberger (Eds.), *Changing patterns in residential services for the mentally retarded* (pp. 227-254).

Beck-Ford, V. (1981). Leisure training with developmentally handicapped adults. In P. Mittler (Ed.), *Frontiers of knowledge in mental retardation: Volume 1. Social, educational, and behavioral aspects* (pp. 255-261). Baltimore: University Park Press.

Bajaanes, A. T., Butler, E. W., & Kelly, B. R. (1981). Placement type and client functional level as factors in provision of services aimed at increasing adjustment. In R. H. Bruininks, C. E. Meyers, B. B. Sigford, & K. C. Lakin, (Eds.), *Deinstitutionalization and community adjustment of mentally retarded people* (pp. 337-350). Washington, DC: American Association on Mental Deficiency.

Blake, R. (1981). Disabled older persons: A demographic analysis. *Journal of Rehabilitation, 47*(4), 19-27.

Developmental Disabilities Assistance and Bill of Rights Act as amended by the Developmental Disabilities Assistance and Bill of Rights Act of 1987, Public Law 100-146. Section 102(5).

Halpern A. S., Close, D. W. & Nelson, D. J. (1986). *On my own — the impact of semi-independent living programs for adults with mental retardation.* Baltimore: Paul H. Brookes.

Hawkins, B. A. & Eklund, S. J. (1989). Aging and developmental disabilities: Interagency planning for an emerging population. *Journal of Applied Gerontology, 8*(2), 168-174.

Jacobson, J. W., Sutton, M. & Janicki, M. P. (1985). Demography and characteristics of aging and aged mentally retarded persons. In M. P. Janicki and H. M. Wisniewski (Eds.), *Aging and developmental disabilities: Issues and approaches* (pp. 115-143). Baltimore: Paul H. Brookes.

Janicki, M. P., Seltzer, M. M., & Krauss, M. W. (1987). *Contemporary issues in the aging of persons with mental retardation and other developmental disabilities.* Washington, DC: Data Institute.

Johnson, M. & Olson, L. M. (1982). A guide to alternative programming for older mentally retarded developmentally disabled adults. Project report from the productive living board for the developmentally disabled of St. Louis County, pp. 1-159.

Kauppi, D. R. & Jones, K. C. (1985). The role of the community agency in serving older mentally retarded persons. In M. P. Janicki & H. M. Wisniewski (Eds.), *Aging and developmental disabilities: Issues and approaches* (pp. 403-409). Baltimore: Paul H. Brookes.

Keller, M. J. (1988). Mainstreaming special populations into community recreation programs. Paper presented at the South Carolina Integration Conference, Columbia, South Carolina.

Krauss, M. S. & Erickson, M. (1988). Informal support networks among aging persons with mental retardation: A pilot study. *Mental Retardation, 26*(4), 197-291.

Provencal, J. (1988). Confessions of a community placement optimist. *Impact, 1,* 5-7.

Putnam, J. W., Werder, J. K., & Schleien, S. J. (1985). Leisure and recreation services for handicapped persons. In K. C. Lakin & R. H. Bruininks (Eds.), *Strategies for achieving community integration of developmentally disabled citizens* (pp. 253-274). Baltimore: Paul H. Brookes.

Rancourt, A. M. (1989). Older adults with developmental disabilities/mental retardation: Implications for professional services. *Therapeutic Recreation Journal, 23*(1), 47-57.

Roberto, K. A. & Nelson, R. E., (1989). The developmentally disabled elderly: Concerns of service providers. *Journal of Applied Gerontology, 8*(2), 175-182.

Rose, T. (1986). *Aging and developmental disabilities from A-Z.* College Park, MD: University of Maryland Center on Aging.

Rose, T. & Janicki, M. P. (1986). Older mentally retarded adults: A forgotten population. *Aging Network News, 3*(5), 17-19.

Seltzer, M. M. & Seltzer, G. B. (1985). The elderly mentally retarded: A group in need of service. *Journal of Gerontological Social Work, 8*(3/4), 99-119.

Shanas, E., & Sussman, M. B. (1981). The family in later life: Social structure and social policy. In R. W. Fogel, E. Hatfield, S. B. Kiesler, and E. Shanas (Eds.), *Aging: Stability and change in the family.* New York: Academy Press.

Sison, G.F.P, and Cotton, P.D. (1989). The elderly mentally retarded person: Current perspectives and future direction. *Journal of Applied Gerontology, 8*(2), 151-167.

Stroud, M. & Sutton, E. (1988). *Expanding options for older adults with developmental disabilities: A practical guide to achieving community access.* Baltimore: Paul H. Brookes.

Sylvester, C. (1989). Quality assurance and quality of life: Accounting for the good and healthy life. *Therapeutic Recreation Journal, 23*(2), 7-22.

Taylor, S. J. (1988). Caught in the continuum: A critical analysis of the principle of the least restrictive environment. *The Journal of the Association of the Severely Handicapped, 13*(1), 41-53.

Thurman, E. (1985). *Community senior integration project.* Grand Rapids, MI: Kent Client Services.

Walz, T., Harper, D., & Wilson, J. (1986). The aging developmentally disabled person: A review. *The Gerontologist, 26*(6), 622-629.

Wolfensberger, W. (1972). *The principle of normalization in human services.* Toronto, Canada: National Institute on Mental Retardation.

Chapter 9

Sharing Activities— The Oneida County A.R.C. Cornhill Senior Center Integration Project

Beth Zimpel

SUMMARY. The integration of older persons with developmental disabilities with their non-disabled peers was investigated. The results indicated that the two groups could successfully integrate.

INTRODUCTION

This chapter describes the task of integrating two groups in the community; seniors who attend the Oneida County A.R.C. Day Treatment Program and seniors who are members of the Cornhill Senior Center. The effort took place in the Summer and Fall of 1989. An analysis of the barriers, process, outcome and dynamics of how and why the integration effort has worked are presented.

ONEIDA COUNTY A.R.C.

Oneida County Association for Retarded Citizens (ARC) operates four day treatment sites throughout Oneida County (located in Central New York). Sites are located in Utica, Knoxboro, and

Beth Zimpel, BS, is Independent Living Skills Coordinator at the Utica Site Day Treatment Program and acted as Project Facilitator for the Sharing Activities Program. Ms. Zimpel has had a life-long interest in anthropology, as well as gerontology, and has traveled extensively throughout the world.

131

Rome, for a total certified capacity of 200 program participants. The Oneida County Association for Retarded Citizens is a founding member of the Central New York Network on Aging and Developmental Disabilities. Each program has at least one seniors' component since about 40% of the persons served are elderly.

Generic integration is one of the most important objectives and the current focus of the shared activities effort at the Utica site. The majority of the seniors at this site are retired sheltered workshop employees who remain active in outlook and lifestyle. The success of this project is their story.

CORNHILL SENIOR CENTER

The Cornhill Senior Center was established in 1978 by a group of people interested in forming an organization that would meet the needs for activities and programs for the area seniors. It also serves as a nutrition site and hosts a summer youth program. "You can be young at any age" is the prevailing philosophy at the center. Goals of the center focus on developing socialization for the membership. It also seeks to service the population of that area with a more multi-purpose center. The immediate concern is to have more participation in new programs and, in the attempt, for multiculturalism, to develop deeper ties with ARC. Cornhill Senior Center is funded by United Way, Utica City Grant, Inkind Funding, memberships and fundraisers.

METHODS

One group consists of older persons with developmental disabilities who are program participants in the senior component of the Oneida County Association for Retarded Citizens (A.R.C.) Arnold Avenue Day Treatment Program. Most of the members have retired from sheltered workshops. The second group is composed of members from the Cornhill Senior Center. These members have been integrated into regular and selected A.R.C. activities. The Center's building is a large, one room, ground level structure, totally accessible to persons with physical disabilities. This building also serves as a nutrition site for seniors in the area.

Cornhill Senior Center is located in an inner city neighborhood, undergoing redevelopment. There are more than normal tensions in the area due to social changes. The community, within the recent past, has been faced with such stressors as different ethnic and racial groups moving into a historically middle class section, which has been experiencing property devaluation, poverty and increased crime. As a result, the area has become stigmatized as being unstable, according to a social impact assessment of the area using methods outlined in *Anthropoligical Proxis*, (Wulff and Fiske, 1987).

Combined with these social tensions, members of the Center are also experiencing the effects of aging and all its involvement. The membership at the Center exceeds 1200. However, the attendance varies with the activity that is being offered on any particular day. Those attending are predominantly white females, and only one or two men are generally present. Some days, the Center is nearly empty; however, on the two days of the week that bingo is offered, the attendance is often as high as 80. This finding is consistent with Decker's (1980) work.

Bingo and day trips seem to be the members' primary interest and activity; however, they have expressed an interest in finding other available activities. The women are active and have a self-determined spirit. They have often remarked that they plan to keep busy as long as they remain in good health.

The ARC's goal for elderly individuals with developmental disabilities is to make available, to them, a typical retirement through activities, services and support in the community. This is to be done through successful integration with other senior citizens, and is in keeping with the philosophy of normalization *(Biklen, 1985)*. It also reinforces in a practical, real-life approach, the skills they work on for more independent living in the day treatment program.

Integration for the Center's members gave them more options for activities, both at the Center and the A.R.C., along with personal associations and experiences. Further, the integration facilitated the change from deriving self-worth from working and receiving a paycheck to self-worth from participating in retirement activities and social interaction (Janicki and Wisniewski, 1985).

APPROACH

Prior to any attempts at integration, a coalition of local service agencies assessed the strengths of such a program for each group. This preliminary effort was instrumental to the program's rename *The Newest Minority: The Aging MR/DD Population in Oneida County*, (1988) reports the findings of the coalition.

Education about the advantages of an exchange of activities was offered to the Center's members. The phrase "shared activities" was used in place of the word integration in this program. This eliminated possible misunderstandings about the goals of the program. Staff members felt that learning about each other would break down barriers of stereotypes, prejudice, and fears. The expectations given to the Center's members was that it would be of mutual benefit to both groups, opening horizons for both.

During the initial attempts at integration, there was a distancing on the part of the members toward the older people with developmental disabilities (DO), and the staff of the A.R.C. To enhance the opportunity for adaptability for both groups, certain techniques were used. The number of the A.R.C. seniors visiting the Center was kept to four or less, to prevent the Center's members from feeling invaded or becoming overwhelmed. The A.R.C. participants were, at first, carefully chosen for their independence, sociability, and appropriate behavior. Also, there was always the same A.R.C. staff person present. The other A.R.C. staff and seniors changed or rotated, but the program leadership remained stable for the Center's members. Eventually, as other senior staff became more familiar with the Center's members, this procedure was not necessary.

Overtures of friendship were offered to the Center's members by the A.R.C. staff. This was done in the form of taking their pictures and returning them to the people after they were developed. A big poster was made from one of the pictures depicting some of the Center's members participating in a bocce play-off that both groups were involved in at Butler Lake. Candy and a newspaper were also offered on the bus going and returning from that day trip. These contributions, and similar ones, aided in indicating to the Center's members that the A.R.C. wanted to add to their center in a positive way.

A survey was conducted to explore areas of interest for the future development of shared activities. This survey, taken at the Center by the A.R.C. staff with the approval of the administration and staff at the Center, was completed by a cross-section of the members (about 50 participated). The survey focused on activities the Center members might want to participate in while at the Center. This reinforced to the Center's members that the Center's and the A.R.C.'s goal in developing new programming activities was to enhance their interests.

RESULTS

As the integration process evolved, avoidance behavior by some Center members subsided. At this stage, other members also began encouraging their peers to be friendly and reach out. The Center's administration and staff also encouraged a friendly interaction.

When some of the Center's members started coming to the A.R.C., they also were carefully selected. They were non-controversial, frequent participants at the center, well respected and had shown friendliness to both the Center's members and the A.R.C. seniors. These members were encouraged to invite a friend from the Center. This technique was instrumental in interesting Center members in attending activities at A.R.C. Another necessary ingredient to the process was to assure that members of both sexes and groups were participants in this endeavor. The report of positive experiences the Center's members had at the A.R.C., such as a sing-along, and a flag raising ceremony, soon spread throughout the Center's membership. Center members who had visited the A.R.C. became strong advocates for this shared programming.

While the Cornhill seniors were at the A.R.C., the staff expressed the gratification experienced with working with its developmentally disabled population. They also saw that the A.R.C. had a cheerful, positive atmosphere. It was also obvious to them that high expectations and the supports to reach those expectations were given to all the people the A.R.C. serves.

The A.R.C. staff acted as behavior role models for the Center's seniors in regard to responding to seniors with DD. It soon became apparent to the non-disabled seniors that their needs and interests were no different than the seniors with DD. This process also worked in reverse; when the A.R.C. seniors visited the Center, they had the Center's seniors behavior to model (Biklen, 1985).

It was obvious from the start of this process that transportation for the Center's seniors to attend the A.R.C. activities must be provided by the A.R.C. The facilitator in the sharing of these activities provided the seniors the options of being picked up at the Center or at their home. Convenience for them was always an important aspect. Other considerations were also offered by the facilitator. She extended friendly greetings to the Center's members when she saw them in other public places, such as, church and a grocery store. Learning their names and their individual interests and concerns was a technique used to stimulate a relationship between the Center's members and the A.R.C. seniors and staff.

The A.R.C. staff and seniors did not expect priority treatment, such as getting on the bus first when going on a day trip. Personal space at the Center was an issue and was given consideration by establishing seating and other routines. When older adults with DD first began coming to the center, they were led to a table where they would sit together. The elderly people with DD decided they wanted to be socially involved with the Center's other members and requested to sit with others.

Recently one senior women with DD won a raffle at the Center while attending a going-away party for the Center's director. She graciously accepted the prize and everybody seemed sincerely pleased and happy for her winning. At both sites, there is respect shown for the existing autonomy and priorities at the host agency.

Successful adaptability of both older people with DD and their nondisabled peers was dependent on the staff demonstrating leadership qualities, sensitivity, observing needs, acting in control, and being flexible. The A.R.C. staff needed to monitor situations and find alternatives when situations did not go according to plans. For example, when one of the seniors with DD required toileting assistance minor changes in the Center's policies were made.

As mentioned previously, in the initial attempts at integration there was a distancing on the part of the Center's members and the A.R.C. seniors. However, there were conditions that prevailed to bridge the gap between the distancing attitude and the actual process of integration. Key elements that played a major role in the integration process were as follows:

a. The process took time.
b. The shared activities were regular (two a week on the average) and on a reocurring basis.
c. There was sharing of activities, meals and equipment.
d. Appreciation of simple pleasures was noticed in the A.R.C. seniors on the part of the Center's seniors.
e. The Center's members started becoming the A.R.C.'s senior supports, such as helping them carry their trays at lunch.
f. The Center's seniors gained satisfaction from a caring, helpful and sharing role.
g. Identification and mutual familiarization took place; the seniors from both sites began to recognize each other when activities were shared.
h. Communication for both groups started occurring.
i. Friendships developed.

The Center seniors have shown a tremendous willingness to make friendships and get involved. In the future, it is possible that volunteers could be developed from this network. These volunteers could potentially aid in the development of additional integration programs.

CONCLUSION

Integration of seniors with DD and their nondisabled peers is a slow process. It required emotional, social, mental, and physical changes (Carter & McGoldrick, 1989). The following are some of the prerequisites or approaches that took place to facilitate these changes:

1. The staff at both sites strongly believed in the advantages of this process for both groups; they had as their goal to make integration work.
2. The presence alone of persons with various developmental disabilities in generic services will not result in true integration of the two groups. Staff have to make integration happen; they accomplished this, in a friendly, caring manner, and through assertiveness and even sometimes aggressive involvement. (Examples of this assertiveness might be in asking to sit with a certain group at their table or participating in line dancing.)
3. Emotional investment for both groups of seniors was also paramount in order for this program to serve the needs of all. Both groups may not derive the same rewards from the integration and activities between them; however, it can be just as satisfying to both.
4. Nondisabled older adults needed to understand and to be recognized for the differences they were making in the lives of older adults with DD.
5. Older adults needed to be shown the commonalities among themselves and those with DD.
6. The Center's members needed to understand that equitable, not necessarily equal, support and services are necessary for all people. Those who have greater needs should have greater access to appropriate services and supports (Sidel & Sidel, 1984).
7. Is it necessary that older people, regardless of condition and station in life, be given opportunities to live a life that is self-fulfilling and meaningful? Has this effort at integration helped this end? We have observed the seniors at the Oneida County A.R.C. enjoying more choices now through their participation in this program—which certainly has improved their sense of dignity and participation in the community. Where in the past older adults with DD had to live with few choices available to them, and had little to do with choosing their residence, education, or work, they now have more options for recreation and

association during retirement years. This effort of intergration has improved the quality of life for all older adults and has offered new opportunities and changes to both older adults with DD and nondisabled older people.

REFERENCES

Biklen, Douglas (1985). *Achieving the Complete School: Strategies for Effective Mainstreaming*. New York: Teachers College, Columbia University.

Carter, Betty, and McGoldrick, Monica (1989). *The Changing Family Life Cycle*. Boston: Allyn and Bacon.

Decker, David (1980). *Social Gerontology: An Introduction to the Dynamics of Aging*. Boston: Little, Brown and Company.

Janicki, M.P. and Wisniewski, H.M. (1985). *Aging and Developmental Disabilities: Issues and Approaches*. Baltimore: Paul H. Brookes.

Task Force Report (1988). *The Newest Minority: The Aging MR/DD Population in Oneida County*. The Oneida County MR/DD Task Force Committee: The Institute of Gerontology, Utica College.

Sidel, Victor, and Sidel, Ruth (1984). *Reforming Medicine: Lessons of the Last Quarter Century*. New York: Pantheon Books.

Wulff, Robert and Fiske, Shirley (1987). *Anthropological Proxis: Translating Knowledge into Action*. Boulder: Westview Press.

Chapter 10

Aging, Developmental Disabilities and Leisure:
Policy and Service Delivery Issues

Ted Tedrick

SUMMARY. Adults with mental retardation/developmental disabilities (MR/DD) are becoming more numerous and are reaching older age. A host of challenges face staff and clients in the MR/DD system as aging begins to occur; likewise, staff in the aging services network are being confronted with a "new" participant, one who may be living in a community setting and desirous of integrated activities. Conceptual and service delivery issues are discussed as in the role of retirement and leisure in the lives of older persons with MR/DD. At present the questions surrounding cooperative initiatives involving the MR/DD system and the aging service network are more numerous than are answers.

While the topic of adults with mental retardation or developmental disabilities who are aging has recently begun to receive increased attention in the fields of leisure and aging and therapeutic recreation (Hawkins, 1987; Hawkins & Eklund, 1989; Rancourt, 1989), there exists a history of legislative mandate and policy directive emanating from administrative and scholarly specialists in the mental retardation/developmental disabilities and aging systems (DiGiovanni, 1978; Janicki & MacEachron, 1984; Dickerson, Hamilton, Huber, & Segal, 1979). This policy activity is in re-

---

Ted Tedrick, PhD, is Associate Professor in Recreation and Leisure Studies with the College of Health, Physical Education, Recreation and Dance at Temple University.

141

sponse to growing numbers of older adults with such special needs and in recognition of the failings of the current delivery systems which often times work separately, are organized to deliver services in different ways, and are funded in dissimilar manners. For staff and clients in the mental retardation/developmental disabilities (MR/DD) networks, the following issues are paramount: how best to deal with clients who are aging; what the concept of retirement should mean to adults in their sixties who have spent years in productive activity in sheltered workshops and no longer are capable of this activity; and how can adults with developmental disabilities be integrated into community-based aging programs and services (Ansello & Rose, 1989; Cotten & Laughlin, 1989; Rancourt, 1989).

A delivery system designed to meet the needs of all older adults, on the other hand, must now begin to consider how best to accommodate persons in their fifties or sixties who may be classified as mildly or moderately retarded and live in some type of community residence. Both staff and regular attenders of senior centers are frequently ill-prepared to respond to this "new" type of visitor (Ossofsky, 1989). Attitudinal readjustment, program design, staff training, and inadequate funding are all considerations faced by the aging services system when older participants with developmental disabilities are considered. Clearly, legislation and policy at the national and state levels are calling for increased cooperation between the two systems (Sanchez, 1990). How agencies should interface, how to fund (perhaps cooperative initiatives, here), and how to insure program effectiveness will all be addressed during the decade of the nineties.

Germane to the awareness of greater numbers of older adults with MR/DD who are aging in place is the role that leisure and recreational programming might serve in their lives. Policy makers are seeking "points of intersection" between the aging network and the MR/DD system (Ansello & Rose, 1989); leisure may indeed offer an excellent way to begin to bring the two systems together. The concept of retirement has already arisen as a topic pertinent to many older adults with developmental disabilities who may no longer be able to maintain employment (Cotten & Laughlin, 1989); what lies on the other side, however, is a question few have much experience with. Those with a background in leisure and aging ought to be able to help conceptualize retirement for an aging developmentally disabled population. "Retirement to" seems a very pressing issue, while "retirement from" has often been the starting point in a society based upon productive and status-oriented employment. Appropriateness of activities during the later years is a further issue of concern when one considers that many mildly retarded older adults live in a community setting where the age range of fellow housemates may be quite large. Thus, the issue of leisure in the lives of mentally retarded or developmentally disabled adults who are aging is one which must be addressed.

This paper will first explore the problems currently seen in defining "developmental disability" when the concept of "aging" is added. Further, the difficulties in assessing how many of these adults exist will be discussed. Recent policy initiatives at the federal and state levels will be reviewed as they pertain to the service delivery systems in both the MR/DD and aging networks. Retirement and leisure will be addressed as specific concerns.

DEFINITIONAL AND DEMOGRAPHIC ISSUES

Perhaps the most widely accepted definition of developmental disabilities stems from 1987 legislation, The Developmental Disabilities Assistance and Bill of Rights Amendment, P.L. 100-146 (see Smoyer & Pappas, 1989, p. 2). It defines developmental disability as "a severe, chronic disability of a person which":

> is attributable to a mental or physical impairment or a combination of mental and physical impairments; is manifested before the person attains age twenty-two; is likely to continue indefinitely; results in substantial functional limitation in three or more of these areas of major life activity: self-care, receptive and expressive language, learning, mobility, self-direction, capacity for independent living, economic self-sufficiency; and reflects the person's need for a combination and sequence of special interdisciplinary, or generic care, treatment, or other services which are of lifelong or extended duration and individually planned and coordinated.

Further, Walz, Harper, and Wilson (1986) noted that mental retardation, cerebral palsy, autism, and other handicapping conditions are considered developmental disabilities and each condition experienced by an adult brings a different set of problems when the aging process advances in adulthood. Mortality rates, cognitive functioning, and causes of death all vary based upon the specific disability. The condition of mental retardation (IQ of approximately 70 or below) is responsible for the largest category of persons with developmental disabilities and Seltzer (1989) indicates that the percentage of persons afflicted differs by age group. Because of less official scrutiny about 1% of adults are classified as mentally retarded while the percentage for school age children is roughly 3%. Furthermore, some older adults may re-enter the MR system after holding jobs and living semi-independently when older age diminishes their functional abilities (Seltzer, 1989).

The issue of establishing a precise year when one with MR/DD becomes "aged" is also a complex issue when individuals and the service system are considered. The heterogeneity of the aging population is a long-held axiom from the field of gerontology. Applied to the aging process the principle sees individuals progressing at different rates when biological, psychological, and functional measures or needs are of concern. Aging for the older developmentally disabled population is much better operationalized at the personal level, yet policy makers and service providers frequently approach the eligibility issue with a specific chronological age serving as a demarcation line (Seltzer, 1989).

Experts have acknowledged the problem. The normative-statistical approach related to signs and symptoms or decline is currently in use (Walz, Harper, Wilson, 1986). Dickerson et al. (1979) indicated that social expectations for those with developmental disabilities may begin to change as early as 35. Others see the mid-fifties as appropriate (Janicki et al., 1985). Both Down's Syndrome and cerebral palsy are known to create debilitating effects associated with aging such that the thirties or forties might be considered appropriate as a late-life stage (Thase, 1982; Janicki and MacEachron, 1984). Seltzer (1989) points to the ages of 60, 62, or 65 as commonly associated with aging while 55 has been used as a lower limit with MR/DD populations. Clearly, this issue is one which must be resolved if clients are to benefit and the MR/DD and aging services systems are to cooperate in the future. An inflexible, age-specific criterion used for eligibility must be balanced against the personal needs of adults with varying types of developmental disabilities.

Similar to definitional issues, there is also little consensus as to how many older adults with life-long developmental disabilities exist. Living situations vary widely and it is estimated that many adults with DD are now living in a two generational aging family, their parents perhaps in the late seventies or early eighties, and the older children may have never had contact with MR/DD or aging services networks. Rose and Linz (1987) estimate the total MR/DD population as somewhere between 200,000 and 500,000 older persons. In 1985, Medicaid counted 146,000 older residents in intermediate care facilities for the mentally retarded and Health Care Financing Administration figures showed 140,000 mentally retarded persons in nursing homes during the same year (Rose and Linz, 1987). The latter report further indicated that few of the group were receiving the developmental services they needed. Walz, Harper, and Wilson (1986) analyzed the prevalence issue and concluded that most projections are based on using a certain percentage and applying that to the total population above 55, or 60, or whatever age is used to define "older." The studies reviewed varied widely as to the percentages used and the authors used a figure of roughly 200,000 older adults with MR in the early 1980's. Most studies further revealed that very few persons are actually receiving services. Seltzer (1989) suggests that the 1% prevalence rate is a crude measure and that only 40% of the older mentally retarded population is known to the service network. Thus, while estimates of this population are questionable in terms of accuracy, more disheartening is the gap which exists between persons in need and the service network.

Finally, mention should also be made of the situation faced by those older adults with chronic disabilities who are borderline cases yet may not qualify for any type of developmental or aging service. They may be a bit too young or have a problem not quite severe enough to qualify for assistance. Yet, their daily living pattern may be one filled with constraints and barriers. Research on poverty in old age has revealed a large group to exist just on the fringe of the cutoff point for annual income (Cook & Kramek, 1986; Uehara, Geron, & Beeman, 1986). For this group, lack of income presents daily struggles, but their numbers aren't counted in official statistics. So, too, with many elderly adults suffering from chronic disabilities. They may be barely ineligible for services, but daily living presents extreme challenges. This situation would suggest using measures of functional ability as key determinants in deciding who may receive assistance.

POLICY INITIATIVES

A major impact of recent legislation and policy directive of the MR/DD and aging services delivery systems has been the emphasis upon formal linkages and initiatives to bring about greater cooperation between the two networks (Sanchez, 1990; Ossofsky, 1989; Ansello and Rose, 1989). A greater awareness of the pertinent issues has been the result of legislation and policy meetings of administrators and field staff in the MR/DD and aging networks (Sanchez, 1990). Funding for research and demonstration projects (See *Staff, Aging and Research Training News*, Feb. 12, 1990) has also been allocated for investigation into the effects of aging upon adults with developmental disabilities.

Recent federal legislation has brought the issue of disability and aging to the fore. In September, 1989, The Senate passed the "Americans With Disabilities Act" (Associated Press, 1989) and the House of Representatives was scheduled to vote on the bill (H.R. 2273) in May of 1990. Its passage would establish a tone of nondiscrimination and equal access for Americans with disabilities. The 1987 Developmental Disabilities Assistance and Bill of Rights Amendment addressed unserved populations (among them the elderly) and provided for much needed training for professionals in the MR/DD and aging systems (Smoyer & Pappas, 1989). In the early 1970's, University Affiliated Programs (UAP's) were funded to provide interdisciplinary training, technical assistance, demonstration projects, research, and dissemination of material about developmental disabilities. Currently funded are 8 UAP's dealing specifically with DD and aging. Located at the University of Georgia, Indiana, Missouri at Kansas City, Montana, Rochester, and Wisconsin, and at the Shiver Center in Massachusetts and the University of Miami School of Medicine, these programs are engaged in serving clients at clinics, integrating clients into the aging network, developing training materials (the program at Indiana has created a module on leisure) and sharing information with practitioners and researchers (Seltzer and Davidson, 1989).

Requests for proposals from federal agencies have focused upon developmental disabilities and aging. The National Institute on Aging has called for proposals on the social, psychological and biological aspects of aging in retarded adults (See *Staff, Aging and Research News*, Jan. 1, 1990). Likewise, the Administration on Aging is preparing to fund three projects at the state level which will bring about greater involvement of the aging network and the DD system (*Staff, Aging and Research Training News*, Feb. 12, 1990). Activity such as this will support the pure and applied research which is so needed currently.

Conferences and symposia have also begun to create an awareness of the need to assist those with lifelong developmental disabilities. The Wingspread Conference held in June of 1987 brought together an elite group of specialists in MR/DD and aging and provided an opportunity for state level planners in both areas to discuss issues central to each and to explore avenues of cooperation (Ansello and Rose, 1989). A regional conference "Aging and Disabilities: Developing a New Partnership" held in January, 1990 in Philadelphia stressed cooperation, cross-cutting issues, and topic sessions ranging from nutrition to family issues to leisure as a point of intersection. The 1989 Congress of the National Recreation and Park Association featured a workshop entitled "Leisure and Aging with Persons who have Disabilities." This special edition of *Activities, Adaptation, and Aging* further exemplifies that MR/DD and aging concerns must be addressed and that leisure or recreational activities offer an appropriate vehicle for merging the strengths of staff in both systems to benefit older participants.

DELIVERY SYSTEM ISSUES

Similar to the definitional and prevalence problems mentioned earlier, the pathway to a cooperative delivery system serving older adults with developmental disabilities is progressing at a rather uneven pace. Foremost among the difficulties are the differences in intent, organizational structure, and reimbursement or funding patterns of the two service systems. Clark (1988) noted that the DD/ MR system is client-driven with agencies receiving funds based upon individual client-care needs. The purpose is to provide for total care and there is a notable medical model emphasis in treatment. The ratio of staff to clients may approach 1:1. Medicaid is a prime reimbursement source.

The generic aging services network on the other hand, is program-driven (the various "Title" programs at the federal level) and often focuses upon serving groups under a given category. The ratio of staff to clients is typically higher than in the MR system. Less individual treatment and fewer prescriptive measures exist within generic aging services. Funding most often is received under program categories.

With these dissimilarities in existence cooperative planning must begin if progress is to be made. Who will take the lead, how will staff training needs (a recognition about aging from the MR/DD side and knowledge about disability and its effects from the aging side) be met, and what role might recreation or leisure play as a component of service, are just the beginning of the issues to be explored. When service dollars are at stake it can also be expected that agencies will protect their "turf." If the intent of the previously mentioned federal and state legislation is backed by dollars which call for cooperative program efforts to serve MR/DD persons who are now aged, then the level of tension may be reduced. Clark (1988) has suggested that the aging network be viewed as an appropriate referral source for retirement and recreation activities with funding for such services coming from the MR system. Of course, the above assumes that older participants and staff are prepared to integrate the older person with MR or DD into the activities at the site.

It is also appropriate to speculate on the role that community-based leisure service organizations should assume in attracting this new client. While therapeutic recreation agencies serving community populations are perhaps positioned best to lend assistance, there should also be a response on the part of public parks and recreation departments whose charge is to serve all. Integration should be one of the goals these latter departments are moving toward. The lack of a therapeutic expertise must not deter administrators from entering the networking process; aligned with the knowledge provided by staff from the aging network and with the help of those who assist developmentally disabled persons, recreation professionals can bring their expertise to create leisure opportunities for the MR/DD participant in advanced adulthood. Local government recreation departments have recognized a growing older population; 2/3 offer programs for senior citizens (McDonald and Cordell, 1988). Children and adults with mental retardation or learning disabilities are served at a much lower rate than are senior citizens by public recreation providers (McDonald and Cordell, 1988, pp. 77,80). While not determined by the McDonald and Cordell survey, one could estimate that far, far fewer *aged* adults with mental retardation are engaged in programs offered through public recreation entities.

Planning efforts to better serve adults with developmental disabilities who are aging are to be considered in their infancy, and are becoming increasingly more active. Questions and issues are being raised and this dialogue will hopefully lead to demonstration projects and model cooperative programs. What role leisure will play in these efforts remains to be seen; but programs focusing on meaningful free time activities offer an excellent avenue to bring staff members (aging, MR/DD, and leisure services) together.

RETIREMENT AND LEISURE

The issue of retirement, its meaning, its appropriateness, and its relationship to the practical day-to-day concerns of what to do and how to fill time, has already surfaced as little-explored yet potentially crucial circumstance for the MR/DD adult who is beyond middle age. This author has conducted workshops where staff have discussed the concept of retirement for adults with developmental disabilities. Retirement may prove to be just as crucial for this population as it is for powerful executives. Cotten and Laughlin (1989) have found negative attitudes toward retirement on behalf of some adults with retardation. Like others, this group may be expected to view retirement in a more positive vein when options are discussed and suitable activities are in place.

The issues of later life faced by all older adults seem appropriate for those with developmental disabilities. Will role loss and replacement occur? Does disengagement take on new meaning in lives where withdrawal may have been the norm due to a reluctance on the part of society at large? How important is structure in later life? Hopefully empirical research and analyses of case histories will provide some answers.

From a philosophical perspective might we conceive of retirement as a bridge "to" something rather than a departure from something? The ability to choose is a way of demonstrating power throughout life. Opportunities for choice need to be structured for older adults with developmental disabilities. While not attempting to gloss over the problems of retirement (the loss of status for a group of persons who have spent their lives seeking acceptance , for example) it seems prudent to focus on the opportunities available and to emphasize growth during one's fifties, sixties, and beyond.

A task facing both staff and older DD clients is to take full advantage of the potential of leisure in later life. With non-disabled populations satisfaction and involvement with activities during retirement has been shown to predict satisfaction with life in general (Russell, 1987; Larson, 1978). Leisure also provides a point of intersection for staff and participants. Integration of various groups may occur at leisure settings and planning may commence when the aging, MR/DD, and recreation systems come together. Leisure services professionals and therapeutic recreation specialists in conjunction with staff serving older adults or persons with developmental disabilities can provide a starting point to explore the issues of meaningful retirement for a group of persons with little experience in seeking later life satisfaction. What to choose, how to program and with whom, and what skills staff will need are just a few of the questions in need of answers. Pre-retirement programs need to be structured (Cotten and Laughlin, 1989) to assist the developmentally challenged who are aging and becoming more numerous.

CONCLUSION

The purpose of this chapter was to explore selected issues about aging, developmental disabilities, how services are delivered and what role retirement and leisure might assume in later life. It is heartening to see the emphasis given the topics at the legislative and policy-making levels; it is frightening to recognize the need and combine that with the lack of knowledge we currently have. Advances in knowledge are necessary to begin theory building translated to effective program design. The list of topics not explored here, yet vital to the future, could be a lengthy one. How best to train professional staff is a very pressing concern.

Could a challenge be issued to assemble practitioners, researchers, educators, and policy makers with an interest in leisure and draw upon the knowledge and experiences of those who work with the older MR/DD population for the purpose of seeking answers to the issues raised herein? This special edition is an excellent forum; might we proceed further?

REFERENCES

Ansello, E. & Rose, T. (1989). *Aging and Lifelong Disabilities: Partnership for the Twenty-First Century. The Wingspread Conference Report.* Palm Springs, California: Elder Press.

Associated Press. (1989, October 13). Support for bill on disabled. *The Philadelphia Inquirer*, p. 10A.

Clark, S. (1988, September-October). Persons with lifelong disabilities: Room in the aging network? A view from the aging system. *Perspective on Aging*, pp. 13, 22.

Cook, F. & Kramek, L. (1986). Measuring economic hardship among older Americans. *The Gerontologist, 26*, (1), 38-47.

Cotten, P. & Laughlin, C. (1989). Retirement: A new career. American Association on Mental Retardation, *Aging/MR Interest Group Newsletter, 3*, (3), 13.

Dickerson, M., Hamilton, J., Huber, R., & Segal, R. (1979). The aged mentally retarded: The invisible client, a challenge to the community. In D.P. Sweeney and T.V. Wilson (Eds.), *Double Jeopardy: The plight of aging and aged developmentally disabled persons in Mid-America.* Ann Arbor: University of Michigan, Institute for the Study of Mental Retardation and Related Disabilities.

DiGiovanni, L. (1978). The elderly retarded: A little known group. *The Gerontologist, 18*, 262-266.

Hawkins, B. (1987). Aging and developmental disability: New horizons for therapeutic recreation. *Journal of Expanding Horizons in Therapeutic Recreation, 2* (2), 42-46.

Hawkins, B.A., & Eklund, S.J. (1989). Aging and developmental disabilities: Interagency planning for an emerging population. *The Journal of Applied Gerontology, 8* (2), 168-174.

Janicki, M. & MacEachron, A. (1984). Residential, health, and social service needs of elderly developmentally disabled persons. *The Gerontologist, 24*, 128-137.

Janicki, M., Otis, J., Puccio, P., Rettig, J., & Jacobson, J. (1985). Service needs among older developmentally disabled persons. In M. Janicki and H. Wisniewski (Eds), *Aging and developmental disabilities, issues and approaches.* Baltimore: Paul H. Brooks.

Larson, R. (1978). Thirty years of research on the subjective well-being of older Americans. *Journal of Gerontology,* 33 (1), 109-125.

McDonald, B. & Cordell, H. (1988). Local Opportunities for Americans: Final Report of the Municipal and County Park and Recreation Study. Alexandria, VA: National Recreation and Park Association., pp. 77, 80.

Ossofsky, J. (1989). The aging developmentally disabled as a dimension of all our goals. In E. Ansello and T. Rose, Eds., *Aging and Lifelong Disabilities: Partnership for the Twenty-First Century.* Palm Springs, California: Elder Press, pp. 17-22.

Rancourt, A. (1989). Older adults with developmental disabilities/mental retardation: Implications for professional services. *Therapeutic Recreation Journal,* 23 (1), 47-57.

Rose, T. & Linz, J. (1987, September). Developmental disabilities: Opportunities in LTC. *Contemporary Long Term Care,* pp. 102-103.

Russell, R. (1987). The relative contribution of recreation satisfaction and activity participation to the life satisfaction of retirees. *Journal of Leisure Research, 19* (4), 273-283.

Sanchez, R. (1990, January). Building partnerships between public and private sectors. Presentation at Aging and Disabilities: Developing a New Partnership, Philadelphia.

Seltzer, M. (1989). Introduction to Aging and Lifelong Disabilities: Content for Decision-Making. In E. Ansello and T. Rose, Eds., *Aging and Lifelong Disabilities: Partnership for the Twenty-First Century.* Palms Springs, California: Elder Press, pp. 23-27.

Seltzer, M. & Davidson, P. (1989). Report of the aging iniative task force of the American Association of University Affiliated Programs. In Training Iniative Projects, Annual Report, Fiscal Year 1989. Silver Spring, Md.: American Association of University Affiliated Programs.

Smoyer, D. & Pappas, V. (1989). National Information and Reporting System, 1988 Report. University Affiliated Programs. Silver Spring, Md.: American Association of United Affiliated Programs for Persons with Developmental Disabilities.

Staff. (1990, February 12). AOA applications due April 25, alternatives to institutional care, *Aging and Research Training News,* p. 22.

Staff. (1990, January 1). Research, training and demonstration opportunities: NIA/Aging in the Retarded, *Aging and Research Training News,* p. 5.

Thase, M. (1982). Longevity and Mortality in Down's Syndrome. *Journal of Mental Deficiency Research,* 27, 133-142.

Uehara, E., Geron, S. & Beeman, S. (1986). The elderly poor in the Reagan era. *The Gerontologist,* 26 (1), 48-55.

Walz, T., Harper, D. and Wilson, J. (1986). The aging developmentally disabled person: A review. *The Gerontologist,* 26 (6), 622-629.

BOOK REVIEWS

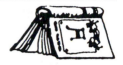

THE WIT TO WIN: HOW TO INTEGRATE OLDER PERSONS WITH DEVELOPMENTAL DISABILITIES INTO COMMUNITY AGING PROGRAMS. Philip LePore and Matthew P. Janicki. *New York State Office for the Aging, 1990, pp. 76.* (For a copy contact: New York State Office for the Aging, 2 Empire State Plaza, Albany, NY 12223-0001.)

In the past, it has been difficult to locate resources that are relevant and helpful in the area of integration of older persons with developmental disabilities (DD). *The Wit To Win: How To Integrate Older Persons With Developmental Disabilities Into Community Aging Programs* is well-written and very readable. The manual discusses the collaboration of three agencies in New York, the State Office for the Aging, Office of Mental Retardation and Developmental Disabilities, and the State Developmental Disabilities Planning Council, to work together under the basic assumption that elderly persons with DD have the right to participate in programs for aging adults and the right to be integrated. Each individual with DD also has a right to receive services in the least restrictive environment and in a way that recognizes that individual's ability to benefit from participation.

This text is an excellent guide for persons providing services to people who are aging and developmentally disabled. The manual explains ways to assist elderly persons with DD to locate and use community programs for elderly people such as senior centers, nutrition sites, and adult day care programs. The manual highlights methods of site selection for older adults with DD; identifies advantages and disadvantages of various aging programs for persons with DD; and explains how both aging and disability service systems are operated and funded. Barriers to integration and formulated strategies to overcome these barriers are addressed.

The text is a useful resource for service providers in aging and developmental disability service systems in regard to collaborating and integrating programs and services. An excellent step by step approach on how to implement an integration program for older persons with DD into community aging programs is introduced. Other agencies in New York as well as in other states can benefit from the model and strategies illustrated. Community programs and their therapeutic values with older adults with DD are outlined. Possibly, the best way to summarize the manual is with the words of Edwin Markham,

> He drew a circle that shut me out —
> Heretic, rebel, a thing to flout.
> But Love and I had the wit to win:
> We drew a circle that took him in!
>
> — Edwin Markham, *OUTWITTED*

Susan E. Lynch, MS
Therapeutic Recreation
Texas Women's University

OLDER ADULTS WITH DEVELOPMENTAL DISABILITIES: AN INTERDISCIPLINARY APPROACH TO GROUPING FOR SERVICE PROVISION. Richard J. Coelho and Norma F. Dillon. *Western Reserve Geriatric Education Center, 1990, 60 pp., $5.00.* (Copies of the text: The Western Reserve Geriatric Education Center, Case Western Reserve University School of Medicine, 12200 Fairhill Road, Cleveland, OH 44120.)

Older Adults With Developmental Disabilities: An Interdisciplinary Approach To Grouping For Service Provision is a valuable resource in familiarizing the reader with the growing population of persons who are elderly and developmentally disabled (DD). The purpose of the monograph is to present the findings of an extensive, interdisciplinary study which delineated the characteristics, service needs, and projected groupings of older adults served by a community based mental health board in Michigan.

The monograph, which was written to expand the knowledge base of service providers who work with older adults with DD, is divided into five chapters: an overview of developmental disabilities; older persons with developmental disabilities; description of the study; results; and discussions and recommendations. Researchers, service planners, and clinicians will find the empirically-derived typology of service needs of developmentally disabled elderly an interesting study with useful implications. The recommendations presented may be helpful in program development and service delivery.

While the study was well outlined, the categorizing and typing of individuals into eight groups were not clearly defined. The authors mixed behavioral assessments with service needs in some cases but not all. Broad generalizations from the study were made; yet, a very small sample which was geographic specific was used. The data regarding needs were compiled through observation rather than any actual input from the sample. Four areas of service were assessed including case management, nursing, day programs, and residential. These four areas may have limited the opportunity to present complete and reliable information of all facets of clients' needs.

The study is a good beginning of data compilation in hopes other communities will likewise gather data about their older population with DD, so that geneneralizations can be made regarding service and program needs and interests of this growing population. The comprehensive model for service delivery supported a need for leisure and activity programming with older adults with DD. The authors challenge human service providers to " . . . expand growth of future services for elderly persons with developmental disabilities." The study also indicated the importance of service providers to act as both suppliers of needed services and advocates for older adults with DD.

Susan E. Lynch, MS
Therapeutic Recreation
Texas Women's University